GUIDE TO OBSERVANCE OF JEWISH LAW IN A HOSPITAL

מדריך לחולים
הנמצאים בבית החולים

RABBI JASON WEINER

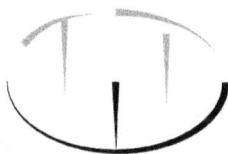

KODESH PRESS, NEW YORK

Kodesh Press is pleased to make *Guide to Observance of Jewish Law in a Hospital* available commercially. It was originally published by the author under the title, *Guide to Traditional Jewish Observance in a Hospital*. The self-published version included additional information specific for the author's hospital, Cedars-Sinai Medical Center, in Los Angeles, California. In the commercial version, those passages have been removed, and some of the material has been rewritten in a more generic manner. No *halachic* material has been altered in any way from the original version for which the accompanying endorsements were written.

Cover Art: Part of the "Jewish Contributions to Medicine" mural by Terry Schoonhover, commissioned for Cedars-Sinai and on permanent display in the Harvey Morse Auditorium. Courtesy of Cedars-Sinai.

Published & Distributed by
Kodesh Press L.L.C.
New York, NY
www.KodeshPress.com
KodeshPress@gmail.com

Table of Contents

All contents of this work have been carefully reviewed by:

Rabbi Gershon Bess שליט״א
Rav of Congregation Kehillas Yaakov & Chaver Beit Din of the Rabbinical Council of California

Rabbi Nachum Sauer שליט״א
Yeshiva of Los Angeles, Dayan & Chaver Beit Din of the Rabbinical Council of California

Rabbi Yosef Y. Shusterman שליט״א
Rav of Chabad of Beverly Hills & Member of the Beit Din of the Vaad Rabbonim Lubavitch

אשר זעליג וייס
כגן 8
פעיה"ק ירושלם ת"ו

בס"ד

תאריך ___ י"ג מרחשון ___

הן ראיתי אשר אמר את הקונטרס היקר ונחוץ מדריך לחולים בלשון האנגלית למחבר הרה"ג ר' יהודה ליב וינר שליט"א, אשר זוכה זה ... את הרב המחבר שליט"א ... מתוארת פעולותיו בבית החולים היקר בלוס אנג'לס ... דבר יום ביומו ואין ערוך לחשיבות פעולותיו.

ועתה הגדיל לעשות קונטרס זה שהוא מדריך לכל דיני חולה בבית החולים. לא הספקתי לעבור על כל הקונטרס אך גדולי הרבנים בלוס אנג'לס כבר העידו על טיבו ושאפשר לסמוך עליו, וכך ...

ברכתי להרה"ג ר' יהודה ליב לכאן חביב נאהב ... ולהאדירה ולקדש שם שמים.

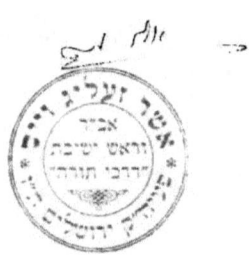

הן ראיתי את הקונטרס היקר והנחוץ מדריך לחולים בלשון האנגלית למחבר ידי"נ האברך הנפלא הרה"ג ר' יהודה ליב וינר שליט"א. מכיר אני זה שנים את הרב המחבר שליט"א ואת יקר תפארת פעולותיו בבית החולים היקר בלוס אנג'לס. הרב וינר זוכה לקדש שם שמים דבר יום ביומו ואין ערוך לחשיבות פעולותיו.

ועתה הגדיל לעשות בקונטרס זה שהוא מדריך לכל דיני חולה בבית החולים. לא הספקתי לעבור על כל הקונטרס אך גדולי הרבנים בלוס אנג'לס כבר העידו על טיבו ושאפשר לסמוך עליו, וכך התרשמתי במעט עיוני בו.

ברכתי להרה"ג ר' יהודה ליב שיזכה תמיד להגדיל תורה ולהאדירה ולקדש שם שמים.

באהבה
אשר וייס

RABBI Yitzchok M.Weinberg
Tolner Rebby

10 David Chazan st.
Jerusalem . Israel

יצחק מנחם ויינברג
נכד אדמו"ר מטאלנא זצללה"ה

רחוב דוד חזן 10
בעיה"ק ירושלים תובב"א

טלפון: Tel. 02-5825543

ב"ה, יום ___ ה' ___ סיון התשנ"א ___

כבוד הרה"ג ר' יהודה לייב ווינער נ"י העוסק בצרכי ציבור באמונה ומרבה להיטיב עם חולי עמך בית ישראל בכל עת ובכל שעה במאור פנים ובשמחה תמיד.

שלו' וברכה

קיבלתי את הקונטרס המיוחד אשר כשמו כן הוא "מדריך לחולים הנמצאים בבית חולים" ועברתי עליו מקופיא ולפענ"ד לענין הלכה למעשה נצרך לקבל עליו הסכמה מפוסק מוכר ומקובל על הכל שיתן חוות דעתו על כל הנכתב ואני מצדי אכתוב הנראה לעניות דעתי.

עצם החוברת וההתייחסות כמעט לכל מצב באופן כ"כ מסודר וברור ובקיצור הוא באמת מפליא לעשות ובטוחני שהמסתייעים מחוברת הזאת ימצאו תועלת מרובה ובזכותה יימנעו מעשרות מכשולים הנמצאים במקומות כאלו לפני כאו"א מידי יום ביומו ע"כ דבר גדול נעשה בזה הראוי לכל שבח ותהילה וזכות שמירת ההלכה במקום זה תעמוד לחולים להירפא במהרה ולקרובי החולים הסועדים אותם והמבקרים שלו' יחילו ולעומד בראש המפעל הקדוש הזה ייאמר לך בכחך ועשה חיל בהבאת דבר ה' זו הלכה למקום שאין בו איש שכרך הרבה מאד ומן השמים יברכוך בכל הברכות ובכפל כפליים.

הכו"ח באהבה ובהתרגשות

בס"ד

RABBI ELAZAR R. MUSKIN
הרב אלעזר ראובן מוסקין

ה' אלול, תשע"ב
August 23, 2012

It is my honor to write this letter of approbation for Rabbi Jason Weiner's work, "Guide to Traditional Jewish Observance in a Hospital."

The Talmud in Megillah 28b states, "It was taught in the Academy of Elijah: Whoever studies Jewish law every day is assured that he will be destined for the world to come." If the Talmud offers this as the reward for one who learns how much more so for one who not only learns Halakha, but also teaches it as well.

Rabbi Weiner is one of those few who not only spends time immersed in the study of Torah and Halakha, but also is a master teacher. I had the honor to work with Rabbi Weiner for three years at Young Israel of Century City where he not only served as the congregation's first Assistant Rabbi, but also became a very dear personal friend. During his tenure, I soon discovered that Rabbi Weiner has an insatiable thirst for knowledge as well as an extraordinary ability to share his love for learning with others. This work is testimony to that ability.

In writing this guide for the Jewish patient, Rabbi Weiner has produced a masterpiece of clarity and organization. I have read the entire work and I am thrilled to endorse it as an excellent addition to the library of Halakhic works that are now being published in English.

May all who use this guide be confident that they are following the letter of the Halakha, and may they receive the divine blessing of a *Refuah Shlema,* a total recovery.

With Torah blessings, I remain,

Elazar Muskin

9500 OAKMORE ROAD • LOS ANGELES, CA 90035 • PHONE: 310/559-9442/9443 • FAX: 310/559-1832 • EMAIL: EMUSKIN@PACBELL.NET
SHUL OFFICE: YOUNG ISRAEL OF CENTURY CITY
9317 WEST PICO BOULEVARD • LOS ANGELES, CA 90035 • PHONE: 310/273-6954 • FAX: 310/273-7103 • EMAIL: SHULOFFICE@YICC.ORG

Iranian Rabbinical
Council of Los Angeles

ربانوت ایرانی مورد تأئید مقام اعظم
ربانوت مرکزی در ارض مقدس

אגוד הרבנים האיראנים
בלוס אנג׳לס
מטעם הרבנות הראשית בארץ

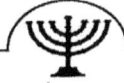

□ כ״ז חשון יום ה׳ לפר׳ ״ומברכך ברוך״ תשע״ב

Nov/ 24/11

הנשר הגדול הרמב״ם מאיר עינים בדבריו בתחילת פ״ג משמונה פרקים וז״ל ״יש לנפש בריאות וחולי כמו שיש לגוף בריאות וחולי״ הרי דעל האדם להשתדל ולשמור על בריאות גוף וגשמיות שלו וכן לשמור על בריאות נפש ורוחניות שלו.

ודא עקא דהרבה פעמים דוקא החולים ורופאים נקלעים בשאלות חמורות ומסובכות וצמאים הם לדבר ה׳ זו הלכה לדעת איזהו דרך הישרה שיבור לו האדם לשמור הגוף גם הנפש ביחד.

והנה קם לעזרם הרב יהודה לייב זוינער רב בבית חולים סידער סיני ועמל וטרח לאסוף וללקוט הלכות בעניינים אלה במדריך הנוכחי למען ירוץ הקורא בו. וסידר הכל בטוב טעם ודעת שימצא בו כל א׳ מבוקשו ויהי׳ כשלחן ערוך ומוכן לפני האדם. ועוד דבר גדול עשה שציין המקורות ג״כ בתוך הקונטרוס למען יהי׳ דבר שלם ומלאכה תמה וכבר סמכו על חיבור זה רבנן מרי חיטיא מורינו הרה״ג בעם שליט״א ומורינו הרה״ג סאווער שליט״א. בודי שהקונטרוס יהי׳ לתועלת גדולה ולזכות הרבים ויקיים על ידי ״וחודעת להם את הדרך ילכו בה ואת המעשה אשר יעשון״ יישר חילי׳ לאורייתא ותהא משכורתו שלמה.

ויה״ר שיפוצו עוד מעינותיו חוצה ותהא משכיל בכל דרכיו ובפרט על עסקו בצרכי הרבים לעודד ולחזק חולים ומשפחותיהם רופא כל בשר יברכהו וישימהו לשליח הגון לרפואת בניו.

ועד הרבנים האיראנים בלוס אנג׳לס

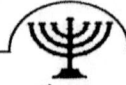

Iranian Rabbinical
Council of Los Angeles

ربانوت ایرانی مورد تأئید مقام اعظم
ربانوت مرکزی در ارض مقدس

אגד הרבנים האיראנים
בלוס אנג'לס
מטעם הרבנות הראשית בארץ

26 חשوان 5762
Nov/ 23/11

هارمبام دانشمند بزرگ یهود در کتاب مشهورش **שמונה פרקים פ"ג** مینویسد: "همانطورکه برای بدن انسان امکان سلامت و بیماری وجود دارد روحانیت وانسانیت فرد نیز میتواند سالم یا خدـای نکرده بیمار باشد." این جملهٔ پر محتوی ما را مسؤل میدارد که چه برای سلامت بدن و چه برای سلامت روحانیت خود با حداکثر توانایی کوشش نماییم.

افراد بیمار و بستری, بسیار مواقع خود را رو در رو با موقعیتهای ناآشنا وجدید میبینند و خواستار آنند که بدانند تصمیم درست واخلاقیِ مورد تائید تورای مقدس چه میباشد. برای کمک به این افراد و همچنین خانوادههایشان "ربای وینر" ربای بیمارستان "سیدر ساینای" با کوشش و پشتکاری زیادشان راهنمایی را که دردست دارید جمع آوری کرده وبه انتشار رسانده اند. در این کتاب, قوانین وهلاخهای مربوطه بصورتی بسیار منظم ترتیب داده شده و منابع اتخاذ نیز ضمیمه شده اند, همچنین این کتاب توسط ربانیم عالیمقام ومرجع تقلید مرورشده ومورد تأیید میباشد.

"ربای وینر" مدائم مشغولِ کمک وبهبودبخشی به بستری شدگان بیمارستان میباشند و یقیناً چاپ وانتشار این جزوه نیزمدد ومساعدت شایان برای بیماران در بر خواهد داشت. از حدـاوند متعال آرزویِ موفقیت وبرکت برای ایشان وهمچنین شفا وسلامتی کا ملِ بیماران داریم.

هیأت ربانوت مقیم کالیفرنیا

Introduction

Purpose

This booklet is designed to assist people observing traditional Jewish Law while undergoing medical treatment, particularly in the complex and unfamiliar environment of a hospital. Patients and families often have a difficult time orienting themselves to unfamiliar circumstances and may encounter questions that they have not previously faced. Furthermore, they may be unable to seek rabbinic counsel (on Shabbat and Festivals for example—the subject of much of this booklet), and are thus in search of guidance. Caregivers also frequently have questions regarding what Jewish Law has to say about patient care and the many issues they face when striving to do what is best for their patients. This booklet is thus shared with medical care providers and used in staff training sessions, but it was written specifically with patients and their visitors in mind.

The idea for this guide emanates from a variety of situations I have witnessed as the Jewish Chaplain at Cedars-Sinai Medical Center in Los Angeles, California. In this position, I have heard stories from both the staff and patients about conflicts that sometimes arise as a result of a patient's desire to observe Jewish Law in the hospital. We have a principle that the Torah's "ways are ways of pleasantness and all its paths are peace" (Proverbs 3:17). The staff wants to respectfully accommodate all patients, and the patients want to carefully observe the laws of their religion in a manner that doesn't agitate anyone and is a sanctification of God's name.

To produce this guide, I have focused on learning about, clarifying, and discussing many situations that are relevant to Jewish observance in a hospital setting. Great effort has also been made to research and present Jewish Law in a manner that is clear, mainstream, and comprehensive.

Guidebooks such as this do exist, but some are very brief and leave numerous questions unanswered, while others are very extensive and thus difficult to utilize when one is ill and when decisions must be made quickly. Therefore, the goal of this work is to examine issues comprehensively and in depth, but without going into excessive detail. Furthermore, since the primary target audience is the hospital patient, I have chosen to address only those issues that commonly arise in a hospital setting. Deciding what to include and what to exclude from this guide was not easy, but based on thousands of patient encounters derived from my professional clinical experience, and with the goal of making this guide comprehensive yet not burdensome, I hope that a happy medium has been achieved.

Methodology

While Jewish Law is very complex and there are numerous opinions about many issues, and variant customs prevail among different communities, this guide seeks to present a mainstream and reliable approach. This goal was achieved by following the rulings of one primary author, complemented by those of other widely accepted authorities where necessary, followed by consultation with local and national rabbinic experts. The school of thought that is followed in this guide has been Professor Abraham S. Abraham M.D., FRCP, author of the "*Nishmat Avraham*," which has become the authoritative medically relevant commentary on the Code of Jewish Law, and "*Lev Avraham*," his digest of rulings relating to patients and their caregivers, which is referenced extensively in this guide. Dr. Abraham quotes primarily from his great teachers, Rav Shlomo Zalman Auerbach, *zt"l*, and Rav Yehoshua Neuwirth *Shlita* (author of the "*Shemirat Shabbat Kehilchatah*"), as well as other leading authorities in Jewish Law. In addition to making careful use of his highly regarded books, Dr. Abraham graciously made himself available for clarifications and specific questions as they arose.

To produce this booklet, I studied each relevant chapter in "*Lev Avraham*," as well as the appropriate related sources, and taught it in the original Hebrew to my weekly *Halachah* (Jewish Law) class at Young Israel of Century City, along with my English summary of each chapter. As a group we discussed the issues, how to present them most clearly, and other relevant questions that may arise. This booklet is the result of one year of these classes.

Acknowledgements

I would like to thank those who regularly attended my weekly classes, and those who read and commented on early drafts of this guidebook, Steve and Rivkie Berger, Rabbi Michael Broyde, Rabbi Daniel Coleman, Rabbi Ari Enkin, Stuart Finder, Ph.D., Chaplain Linda Joy Goldner, Nathaniel Goldstein, Rabbi Avraham Yechiel Hirschman, Rabbi David Hojda, Rabbi Drew Kaplan, Pam Kleinman, Adam and Rachel Lewis, Ben Lipman, Amanda Newstead, Dr. Ronne Penn, Rabbi Dr. Edward Reichman, Elkie Reichman, Rabbi Jackie Siegel, Victoria Shaun, Natasha Somer, Allan Sternberg, Rabbi Mordechai Torczyner, and Rabbi David Wolkenfeld. I would especially like to thank Rabbi Dov Linzer for his insightful comments and suggestions.

I am incredibly indebted to and appreciative of the wonderful local *Rabbonim* who have read and commented extensively on this entire booklet: Rabbi Gershon Bess, Rabbi Elazar Muskin, Rabbi Nachum Sauer, and Rabbi Yosef Shusterman.

A special note of gratitude is also due to Paula Van Gelder, about whom Rabbi Levi Meier Ph.D., *zt"l*, wrote, "her expertise in writing is matched only by her kindness," for not only carefully proof-reading and commenting on every word of this guide, but for assisting me in my research and clarification of hospital policies.

I have the honor of serving as the Senior Rabbi and Manager of the Spiritual Care Department at Cedars-Sinai Medial Center, where so many people, particularly Jonathan Schreiber and the department of Community Relations and Development, have been tremendously gracious, helpful and encouraging of this project.

I am privileged to be able to learn and teach Torah at Young Israel of Century City, under the guidance of Rabbi Elazar Muskin. I would like to thank the *Shul* and Rabbi Muskin for always being so warm, supportive, and interested in learning.

Last but not least, nothing I do would be possible without the incredible blessing of my wife, Lauren, and her tremendous self-sacrifice on behalf of our family and my learning.

Important Note

It is essential to recognize that this booklet is only a guide and an aid, and as such it is not particularly detailed or nuanced. The areas dealt with in this booklet are often very complicated, depend on numerous factors, and are sometimes matters of dispute amongst leading rabbis. **Therefore, it is best to consult with a recognized authority in Jewish Law whenever possible as specific cases arise.**

It is my fervent prayer and deep hope that this guide will serve to facilitate increased observance of Jewish Law and sensitivity to issues that arise in health care settings and that no one will make any mistakes in observing Jewish Law as a result of it. May this guide assist us in creating a *Kiddush Hashem* (sanctification of God's name) wherever we go, and may the Torah learned herein lead to a *Refuah Shelaimah* (complete recovery), as we are taught, "Torah study brings healing for one's body and bones both in this world and in the next" (*Mishnah Berurah* 61:6).

I. Categories of Illness

Jewish Law recognizes five categories of sick patients, each with specific rulings relating to what may be done for that category of patient regarding various issues, such as Shabbat, Passover, fast days and ingesting forbidden foods.

In Case of Emergency

When a person's life is in danger, it is an important *Mitzvah* (religious obligation) to do anything possible to assist them with great speed, as the *Ohr Hachaim* writes, "One who transgresses Shabbat for a dangerously sick person is not called a transgressor of Shabbat, but a guarder of Shabbat."[1] One who hesitates and does not save the person is considered to have shed blood.[2]

A. Minor Ailments

1. **Slight discomfort:** The first category is called a "*Maychush*," which describes someone who is only experiencing slight discomfort that is not severe enough to affect their entire body, such as a runny nose, dry skin or lips,[3] mild cold or cough,[4] minor joint or muscle pains, digestion problems,[5] or a minor toothache.[6] Sabbath and Festival Law may generally not be transgressed for a patient in this category, including the prohibition against taking any form of medication on these days.[7]

2. **Minor Illness:** The second category is called "*Miktzat Choli*" or "*Mitztaer Harbe*" which describes a patient with a minor illness, aches or pains, such as one who is sick and has an irritating cough, headache, or nasal inflammation, which does not affect the entire body or cause a person to be confined to a bed. Jewish Law may generally not be transgressed for a patient in this category either, (including the prohibition against taking medication), though there are certain leniencies, such as the permissibility of asking someone who is not Jewish to perform a labor for them [see **pg. 24**, for an explanation of this concept] if the act is not prohibited by the Torah but only forbidden rabbinically (examples of rabbinic prohibitions are included in **pg. 21**).[8]

B. Incapacitating and Life-Threatening Illnesses

3. **Total body illness:** The third category is known as "*Choleh She'ain Bo Sakana*," which describes a patient who is ill, but not dangerously or seriously ill. Such a patient is one who either has a generalized (systemic) illness, is bedridden (or in a state in which most people would become confined to bed), noticeably not functioning up to par due to pain or illness, but whose life is not in danger.[9]

---

[1] *Ohr Hachaim* Exodus 31:13.
[2] *Shulchan Aruch OH* 328:2, 11-13.
[3] *Lev Avraham* 1:1.
[4] *Shulchan Aruch OH* 328:32.
[5] *Aruch Hashulchan OH* 328:19.
[6] *Shulchan Aruch OH* 328:32.
[7] Ibid., 328:1; *Mishnah Berurah* 328:2-3; *Lev Avraham* 1:1; *Nishmat Avraham OH* 328: Intro (A:2).
[8] Ibid., 307:5; *Mishnah Berurah* 328:52; *Lev Avraham* 1:2; *Shemirat Shabbat Kehilchatah* 34 fn. 7.
[9] Ibid., 328:17; *Lev Avraham* 1:3.

Examples of this category include:

- One whose whole body is affected by illness or pain, such as a moderate fever, influenza (flu), or severe migraine headache.[10]
- One who requires preventive treatment to not become sick, for instance, someone with acute asthma, unless they are receiving preventive treatment.[11]
- One who suffers from chronic debilitating arthritis pain.[12]
- One who suffers from migraine headaches or mild clinical depression.[13]
- A pregnant woman suffering from non-life-threatening complications to her or her fetus (e.g., lower back pain).[14]
- A woman who has given birth in the past thirty days (but not the past week) without any known problems or is experiencing non-life-threatening postpartum complications, in which case this may even apply beyond thirty days after the birth.[15]
- A person with an eye infection, however mild.[16]
- A child up to age nine or ten who has discomfort or even only a mild illness.[17]

Such a patient should carefully follow all of their doctor's instructions. Even if it is not certain if they are sick enough to fall in this category, they should be considered to be in this category and are allowed its following leniencies:[18]

- A patient in this category may request someone who is not Jewish to perform necessary treatments that cannot wait until after Shabbat, even if a Torah prohibition is involved,[19] provided that specific treatment is needed to treat the person immediately on Shabbat.[20]
- Additionally, a Jewish person may do whatever is necessary for the care of such a patient if it involves a rabbinical prohibition (or even a Torah prohibition in a case of great need), if it is done in a manner differing from the way it is ordinarily done [see **pg. 23**, for an explanation of this concept].[21]
- Furthermore, although taking certain medicine and therapeutic treatments are normally forbidden on Shabbat, a patient in this category may take medicine in the normal manner.[22]

---

[10] *Lev Avraham* 1:3.

[11] Ibid.

[12] Rabbi Dovid Heber, "A Kashrus Guide to Medications, Vitamins, and Nutritional Supplements" (based on rulings of Rabbi Moshe Heinemann) *Star-K Kashrus Kurrents*, http://www.star-k.org/kashrus/kk-medi-guide.htm#fA.

[13] Ibid.; Rabbi Yisroel Pinchas Bodner, *Halachos of Refuah on Shabbos*, 43.

[14] Ibid. Pregnancy complications are very complex, and we treat the life of the fetus like a person for these matters.

[15] *Shemirat Shabbat Kehilchatah* 36:15.

[16] Ibid., 34:8.

[17] *Shulchan Aruch OH* 328:17; *Shemirat Shabbat Kehilchatah* 37:2. While opinions vary regarding what age is still considered a "child" for these matters, with some opinions that it is even as old as thirteen, the general rule is that each child should be judged separately based on his or her individual constitution and strength. Others rule that above the age of two or three, a child should no longer be assumed to fit into the category of dangerously ill. Furthermore, if it is possible to help a sick child without violating any transgressions, that is always preferable (See *Nishmat Avraham OH* 328:17 (57)).

[18] *Minchat Shlomo* 2:34 (36).

[19] *Shulchan Aruch OH* 328:17 & *Mishnah Berurah* 328:47.

[20] *Mishnah Berurah* 328:46.

[21] Ibid., 328:57; *Lev Avraham* 1:3; *Nishmat Avraham OH* 328:17 (48).

[22] *Shulchan Aruch OH* 328:37 Rema; *Mishnah Berurah* 328:121.

4. **Limb-Threatening:** The fourth category is where there is a danger of losing or causing permanent significant damage to a limb (*"Sakanat Eiver"*). Someone who is not Jewish may be asked to perform a Torah prohibition for their sake, or a Jewish person may perform a Torah prohibition provided they deviate from the normal weekday manner (*"Shinui"*), or a rabbinic prohibition even in the normal manner.[23] However, if there is a concern that this damage to a limb may lead to more serious danger to the individual, all prohibitions may be suspended.[24] Similarly, to save an eye, or even to prevent blindness, all prohibitions may be suspended.[25]

5a. **Potentially Life-Threatening:** The fifth category is a *"Choleh Sheyaish Bo Sakana"* which describes a patient who is seriously or dangerously ill, suffering from a **potentially** life-threatening condition, even if it is **not certainly** life-threatening,[26] as long as a doctor agrees that there is some danger.[27]

5b. This category includes one whose life is currently not in danger, but if untreated could develop a life-threatening complication, such as an elderly person who has the flu, an infant with a fever, or a diabetic in need of insulin.[28] Moreover, if the patient is in the process of dying, prohibitions may be transgressed to keep them alive even for a few extra minutes.[29]

5c. Many examples and specifics will be discussed below, but some examples of patients who are considered to be in life-threatening danger include:

- One who has a serious heart condition, diabetes, substantially elevated blood pressure, kidney disease, severe depression,[30] or any other serious condition which may potentially be life-threatening.[31]

- Someone with a potentially life-threatening infection may take antibiotics even if it entails violating a Torah prohibition.[32]

- A pregnant woman whose life is in danger (e.g., blood clotting disorder, toxemia), or who is in active labor, or who is in danger of having a miscarriage.[33]

- Very high fever (determined by how the patient feels, but is generally considered very high at approximately 102 degrees for an adult, and even lower for a child).[34]

If actual or possible danger to such a patient's life is imminent, one must do everything necessary to save the patient's life as speedily as possible without

---

[23] *Lev Avraham* 13:20; *Lev Avraham* 1:3 based on *Shulchan Aruch OH* 328:17 & *Mishnah Berurah* 328:57.

[24] *Lev Avraham* 1:3. Nowadays, it is assumed that the entire body of most patients in the category of *"Sakanat Eiver"* is in danger. A Jew may thus violate even Torah prohibitions for such a patient, if necessary (*Nishmat Avraham* OH 328:17 (49) & *Tzitz Eliezer* 8:15 (10:9)).

[25] Ibid.; *Shulchan Aruch OH* 328:9 & *Mishnah Berurah* 328:22.

[26] *Lev Avraham* 1:4; *Shulchan Aruch OH* 328:10-14.

[27] *Shemirat Shabbat Kehilchatah* 32 fn. 25.

[28] *Mishnah Berurah* 328:17; *Shemirat Shabbat Kehilchatah* 32:8; *Lev Avraham* 1:4.

[29] *Shulchan Aruch OH* 329:4.

[30] *Igrot Moshe EH* 1:65.

[31] Star-K Kashrus Kurrents: "A Kashrus Guide to Medications, Vitamins, and Nutritional Supplements" By Rabbi Dovid Heber based on rulings of Rabbi Moshe Heinemann, http://www.star-k.org/kashrus/kk-medi-guide.htm#fA.

[32] Ibid.

[33] Ibid.

[34] *Igrot Moshe OH* 1:129 based on *Shulchan Aruch OH* 328:7.

asking anyone else to do it for them, and on Shabbat it may be done exactly as one would were it not Shabbat.[35] All instructions given by the doctor should be carefully followed, including taking the medication for the prescribed number of days, even though the symptoms may have subsided.[36]

- One whose life is in any sort of danger as a result of mental illness/psychiatric disorder is treated just as seriously as in the case of physical illness.[37]

Summary

Medical Condition	Permitted Response
Potentially Life-Threatening *"Choleh Sheyaish Bo Sakana"* (Possibly seriously or dangerously ill, or may become so)	Minimal restrictions: one must act quickly to ensure that all medical needs are met. A Jew may respond just as he or she would during a weekday, despite violating Torah prohibitions if necessary. All medical instructions must be followed.
Limb-Threatening *"Sakanat Eiver"* (Danger of losing or causing permanent significant damage to a limb)	• May ask someone who is not Jewish to perform any action needed to treat the patient immediately on Shabbat, even if it violates a Torah prohibition. • A Jewish person may do anything necessary to care for this patient (even if it violates a Torah prohibition) as long as it is done in a manner differing from what would be done on a weekday (*"Shinui"*). • A rabbinic prohibition may be violated for this patient even in the normal manner. • If there is concern that this may lead to more serious danger (or to prevent blindness), or if the broken limb may be life-threatening, all prohibitions may be transgressed.
Incapacitating Illness *"Choleh She'ain Bo Sakana"* (bedridden or total body illness – not functioning well but not life threatening)	• May ask someone who is not Jewish to perform any action needed to treat the patient immediately on Shabbat, even if it violates a Torah prohibition. • A Jewish person may do anything necessary to care for this patient if it involves a rabbinic prohibition (or even a Torah prohibition in a case of great need) ideally done in a manner differing from what would be done on a weekday (*"Shinui"*). • May take medicine in normal manner.
Minor Ailment I *"Miktzat Choli"* or *"Mitztaer Harbe"* (minor illness, localized aches/pains)	One may ask a person who is not Jewish to perform only actions that are rabbinically prohibited.
Minor Ailment II *"Maychush"* (slight discomfort)	May not violate any Sabbath restrictions.

---

[35] *Shulchan Aruch OH* 328:2, 5.
[36] Rabbi Dovid Heber, "A Kashrus Guide to Medications, Vitamins, and Nutritional Supplements" (based on rulings of Rabbi Moshe Heinemann) *Star-K Kashrus Kurrents*, http://www.star-k.org/kashrus/kk-medi-guide.htm#fA.
[37] *Nishmat Avraham OH* 328: Intro (6:2).

II. Shabbat

Shabbat is the Jewish Sabbath. It commemorates God's resting from the creation of the universe on the seventh day and is observed by emulating God through ceasing various activities, resulting in a restful and spiritual atmosphere. Shabbat begins before sundown every Friday night and lasts until approximately 45 minutes or more (practices vary) after sundown on Saturday night. <u>Careful and precise fidelity to the intricate rules of Shabbat is of tremendous importance to traditionally observant Jews.</u>

A. Dangerously Ill Patient on Shabbat and Holidays – General Principles

1. Whenever there is any danger to human life, even if it is only possible danger, one is required to set aside the laws of Shabbat and holidays to do everything that is necessary for the benefit of the sick person.[38] The *Mishnah Berurah* states that "If a person is overly pious and fears to desecrate Shabbat for such a patient without first asking a Torah authority, they may be guilty of bloodshed… If the patient is afraid to have people transgress Shabbat for their sake, one must compel them to allow it to be done and set their mind at rest by explaining that the piety of refraining from Shabbat desecration in such a case is mere folly."[39]

2a. When Shabbat is violated in order to save a person's life, it may be done either by the person whose life is in danger or by someone else who is trying to help.[40] If the process of attending to a patient will not be slowed down at all or in any way compromised by performing an action with a "*Shinui*" (obvious change from the normal manner, see **pg. 23**, for an explanation of this concept), that is preferred. If it can be done by asking someone who is not Jewish to do it for them [see **pg. 24**, for an explanation of this concept], such would be preferable.[41] Furthermore, if it is certain that there is no imminent danger to life in taking time to consult a competent authority in Jewish Law, one should do so.[42]

2b. However, **if any of these deviations from the norm will cause the process to be delayed at all or done imperfectly,** in a case where this could put the patient in danger, the action should be done right away by any person—including a Jewish person, and in a normal way, in which case the *Mishnah Berurah* writes, "even if it is doubtful as to whether or not the action will save life but there is definite danger to life involved, whoever is brisk in performing the action with their own hands is worthy of praise, even though they will thereby desecrate Shabbat."[43]

---

[38] *Shulchan Aruch OH* 328:2 & *Mishnah Berurah* 328:6; *Rambam, Hilchot Shabbat* 2:1. This includes violating Torah prohibitions.

[39] *Mishnah Berurah* 328:6.

[40] *Shemirat Shabbat Kehilchatah* 32:4.

[41] *Shulchan Aruch OH* 328:12 *Rema*; *Mishnah Berurah* 328:14; *Lev Avraham* 1:5. However, the *Rambam, Hilchot Shabbat* 2:3 and the *Shulchan Aruch OH* 328:12 rule that we should not ask anyone else to perform the forbidden Shabbat labor, but a Jew must in fact desecrate Shabbat for the sake of the patient.

[42] *Lev Avraham* 1:6.

[43] *Mishnah Berurah* 328:37.

2c. The above applies only to the direct needs of the patient. However procedures which are not absolutely necessary are ideally done by someone who is not Jewish [see **pg. 24**, for an explanation of this concept] or through a "*Shinui*" (obvious change from the normal manner—see **pg. 23**, for an explanation of this concept).[44]

2d. However, if there is an important need for something, even if not directly related to the patient's healing, but to reducing the patient's suffering or strengthening their body, Shabbat should be violated in order to do this.[45]

3. The decision to suspend the laws of Shabbat on behalf of a patient should be made based on what one would do if it was not Shabbat. If the patient was so seriously ill that they would certainly go to the emergency room or call the doctor immediately on a weekday, even in the middle of the night, the same should be done on Shabbat. However, if one would find it medically prudent to wait a few hours or until the next day on a weekday, they must also wait until after Shabbat.[46] On the other hand, even if one would normally attend to their illness right away, but it is clear to them or their doctor that they can safely wait until Shabbat is over to obtain treatments that violate Torah prohibitions without any danger, they should wait until after Shabbat concludes.[47] In such a case, however, it may be permissible to violate rabbinic prohibitions.

4a. Some examples of **rabbinically** forbidden Shabbat actions include:[48]

- "*Muktzeh*": the restrictions on moving certain objects, such as money, electronics, or writing utensils.

- Re-heating solid food on a pre-lit stove.

- A left-handed person writing with their right hand or a right-handed person writing with their left hand [see **pg. 38**, for an explanation of this concept].

- Asking someone who is not Jewish to violate any Torah level prohibition [see **pg. 24**, for an explanation of this concept].

- Preparing on Shabbat for a weekday.

4b. Some examples of activities forbidden by the **Torah** on Shabbat include:[49]

- Starting and driving a car.

- Adjusting the thermostat so that the furnace goes on immediately.

- Turning on an electric or gas oven.

- Boiling a liquid (or even just heating to a temperature hot enough to cause a person to reflectively withdraw their hand).

- Writing with a pencil or pen.

---

[44] *Nishmat Avraham OH* 328:Intro (2).
[45] *Shemirat Shabbat Kehilchatah* 32:22.
[46] *Lev Avraham* 13:4.
[47] *Mishnah Berurah* 328:15 & 46.
[48] Nachman Schachter, *Guide to Halachos*, edited and approved by Rabbi Moshe Heinemann, (Feldheim publishers), 35.
[49] Ibid.

5. A patient who has an incapacitating illness, even though it is certainly not life-threatening, may instruct somebody who is not Jewish to perform medically necessary tasks for them, even if it involves setting aside a Torah prohibition.[50] A Jew may only perform an act which is rabbinically prohibited for such a patient, but if possible doing so in a different manner than usual.[51]

Treatment Options

6. The book "*Shemirat Shabbat Kehilchatah*" states, "A person whose life is regarded as being in danger should be given any treatment required for their recovery, or to prevent worsening of their condition, even if: a) there is only a possibility that their condition will worsen, b) the treatment involves the violation of Shabbat by transgressing a Torah prohibition, c) it is not certain that the action undertaken will indeed help remove or minimize the danger."[52]

7. Even if there are treatment options that do not involve any Shabbat violations, a patient whose life may be in danger may still suspend the Shabbat laws to pursue treatment if it is more effective than the options that do not involve Shabbat violation.[53] For example:

- A patient may call a doctor outside of the hospital, despite the fact that it will involve Shabbat violation, if the doctor who lives far away is more competent, **or** has been treating the patient regularly and knows the medical history better, **or** the patient prefers their own private doctor, assuming they will get more devoted attention.[54]

- If there is a need for a light to be on in the room of a dangerously ill patient, even if light can be brought in from another room, a light may be turned on if their current light is not bright enough, **or** the time delay will endanger the patient.[55]

Fetus & End-of-Life Patient

8. These rules apply equally to an adult, a child, a fetus in any stage of gestation, or a child who will live for only a limited time.[56]

9. These rules also apply to a person who is near the end of life, even if the dying process has begun. The laws of Shabbat and holidays are still suspended in order to help a person live just a short while longer[57] or even to just temporarily relieve suffering.[58]

---

[50] *Shulchan Aruch OH* 328:17, *Mishnah Berurah* 328:47.
[51] Ibid., *Mishnah Berurah* 328:50 & 54.
[52] *Shemirat Shabbat Kehilchatah* 32:18.
[53] Ibid., 32:27.
[54] Ibid., 32:38; *Lev Avraham* 13:14. This does not apply if the only concern is saving money.
[55] Ibid., 32:65.
[56] Ibid., 32:3 fn. 14; *Lev Avraham* 13:8.
[57] *Shulchan Aruch OH* 329:4; *Shemirat Shabbat Kehilchatah* 32:2.
[58] *Lev Avraham* 13:5.

Psychiatric, Dementia, or Suicidal Patient

10.   The same rules governing one who has a physical infirmity apply to one whose life is in danger—or presents a danger to other people's lives—due to a psychiatric condition,[59] or is in danger as a result of a condition such as Alzheimer's disease.[60] Shabbat may be violated for such patients, including Torah prohibitions if necessary, in accordance with the severity of their mental illness. So too, Shabbat must be transgressed to treat a patient who has attempted suicide and thus places him or herself in danger.[61]

B. "Shinui": Doing a Shabbat labor in an awkward, backhanded manner

The concept known as "Shinui," that was previously mentioned, means performing an action which is forbidden on Shabbat in a manner that is irregular and different from the way it is normally done during the week.

The Shabbat prohibitions are based on labors that were performed in the construction of the Tabernacle (Mishkan), as described in the Torah. Since these were skilled labors, an action done with this awkward or backhanded manner does not conform to the character of the precise actions used in the construction of the Tabernacle. Torah law thus only prohibits work done in a normal way. Therefore, when one does an action in an abnormal manner, although it is still forbidden, the level of prohibition is downgraded. If the action is a Torah prohibition, doing it in this abnormal manner reduces it to a rabbinic prohibition. If the action is already a rabbinic prohibition, it becomes a less severe rabbinic prohibition.

The only way to actually make a forbidden action permitted is when it is combined with other mitigating factors. For example, it is permitted to violate a rabbinic Shabbat prohibition in an abnormal manner to assist an individual with an illness which causes one to be bedridden even if non-life-threatening. Further examples include turning on a light in a case where light is needed on Shabbat. One should not turn it on with their fingers in the normal manner, but must instead use something unusual and awkward, such as an elbow.[62] Simply using the left hand in place of the right hand is not a sufficient deviation from the normal way of doing things for most Shabbat violations, with the notable exception of writing.[63]

---

[59]   Ibid., 13:9.
[60]   *Tzitz Eliezer* 8:15 (3:1).
[61]   *Igrot Moshe OH* 1:127.
[62]   *Shulchan Shlomo* 328:28 (2).
[63]   *Chayei Adam, Hilchot Shabbat* 9:2.

C. *"Amira L'Akum"*: Asking someone who is not Jewish to violate Shabbat

Another circumstance in which actions forbidden on Shabbat can be permitted in certain situations is when one asks someone who is not Jewish to do the action for them. This principle should by no means be misinterpreted as any inference of superiority or inferiority between religions. Rather, it is a simple acknowledgement of the fact that people who are not Jewish are not obligated in the laws of the Jewish Sabbath and may, therefore, be helpful to someone who is Jewish by doing things on their behalf. Essentially, this is little different from the myriad ways in which people, of all races and religions, help each other in all spheres of life—including help that allows another to observe his or her religion's demands. Indeed, Judaism **obligates** us to treat people who are not Jewish with kindness and respect and to never behave in a manner towards them that could be perceived as rude or impolite.

It should be pointed out that generally speaking the Sages prohibited a Jew from asking someone who is not Jewish to perform a forbidden Sabbath act on behalf of a Jew.[64] These laws are very complex and detailed, but for our purposes we may simply point out that the Sages waived the restriction of asking someone who is not Jewish in certain specific circumstances, such as to assist in the care of a person who is ill (as detailed above in chapter 1).[65]

Normally, one who is not Jewish may only be asked to do certain forbidden Shabbat labors for a Jew if the non-Jew acts completely on his or her own accord or one hints to the non-Jew in an indirect manner. However, in a case of a person who is ill, even not dangerously so, in most situations one need not hint but may directly ask a person who is not Jewish to do any action for them, and the prohibition to benefit from it is set aside.[66]

If one must violate Jewish law for the sake of a patient, and either option is equally viable, it is generally preferable to ask someone who is not Jewish to perform the action rather than to have someone who is Jewish do it in an abnormal manner.[67]

It is generally best to alert staff members who are not Jewish in advance to any requests that you may make on Shabbat and holidays, sensitively explaining that these are based on religious observance. By doing so, you can help prevent any misunderstandings or misperceptions (such as "Why can't they do that for themselves?"). Also, when you ask someone who is not Jewish to accommodate your special needs, it is essential to speak in a very polite manner, without ever appearing condescending or simply expecting that someone should go out of their way for you. The best approach in all interpersonal relations is to imagine what it is like to stand in the other person's shoes.

---

[64] *Rambam, Mishnah Torah Hilchot Shabbat* 6:1.
[65] *Shulchan Aruch OH* 307:5 & *Mishnah Berurah* 21.
[66] *Shulchan Shlomo, Erchei Refuah*, vol. 1, 47.
[67] *Nishmat Avraham* OH 307:1 (5).

D. Use of Electricity

The activation and deactivation of electrical appliances is forbidden on Shabbat. Therefore, when it is not medically necessary, traditionally observant Jews will refrain from directly activating or deactivating any sort of electric devices, such as lights, televisions, call buttons, or elevators.

While the nature of the prohibition related to the use of electricity on Shabbat is the topic of much debate and various opinions, our approach in this guidebook for people who are ill and hospitalized is to follow Rav Shlomo Zalman Auerbach, who understood the verse "One may not create a fire on Shabbat in all your dwellings" (Exodus 35:3) as explaining the prohibition to use electricity as follows: "fire" is the source of heat and light and therefore turning on any electrical device that produces both heat and light is forbidden by Torah law on Shabbat. For example, incandescent light bulbs and glowing red hot electric heaters are prohibited by Torah Law, but electric lights such as neon, florescent, LED, digital (LCD), or lights which do not emit heat are treated as rabbinic prohibitions, as are electrical appliances that produce mechanical energy without lights, such as a fan, many air conditioners, or an electric door.[68]

In the past, most electric appliances with a light would fall under the Torah prohibition, since that light was usually incandescent and could thus be switched on by a Jew only for a dangerously ill patient (if someone who is not Jewish was not available to do so). At the present time, however, many lights in modern appliances, particularly in a hospital setting, are florescent, LED or neon. These appliances, whose use would thus not be prohibited by the Torah according to most opinions, may be activated for the sake of a patient with an incapacitating illness, even if not dangerously ill (ideally in an abnormal manner). Therefore, the actual rulings may vary from what is written in this section depending on the type of technology being used. One should seek competent rabbinic guidance to determine the status of any given electrical appliance.

Turning Lights On and Off

1a. When there is a sick person whose care may require light, one should turn on a light before Shabbat (preferably just outside their room), so that it will be possible to see well enough to attend to their needs during the night without turning on a light (as long as the light does not disturb them).[69]

1b. However, one may turn on a light on Shabbat for a sick person whose life is in danger, when there is nobody who is not Jewish available:

---

[68] Personal correspondence with Dr. Abraham S. Abraham [see also *Encyclopedia Talmudit* volume 18, pgs. 185 (especially footnote 360), 715 – 716 & Rabbis M. Broyde and H. Jachter, "The Use of Electricity on Shabbat and Yom Tov," *The Journal of Halacha & Contemporary Society*, Vol. 21 (1991), 4-46]. In many places, a more stringent position is taken in this Guidebook in order to be cautious to avoid any possible transgressions. Furthermore, even though some appliances do not fall under the category of Torah prohibitions based on the definition above, there are sometimes other reasons why they are nevertheless not permitted.

[69] *Shemirat Shabbat Kehilchatah* 32:63. See the beginning of this section for further clarification.

- Whenever darkness or poor light hinders one in doing what is required to care for them, **or**

- So that they will not be afraid of the dark, **or**

- To make them feel that they are being taken care of and to avoid their having the impression that they are being neglected or not receiving proper attention, an impression which is liable to have a detrimental effect on their state of health. [70]

2. One may not turn on a light for a patient who has a non-life-threatening serious illness, even in an abnormal manner, though one may ask someone who is not Jewish to turn on a light for such a patient [see **pg. 24**, for an explanation of this concept]. However, a Jew may turn the light off in an abnormal manner (though it is also preferable for someone who is not Jewish to turn the light off, if possible).[71]

How to Turn the Light On

3. If one has to turn on the light for a dangerously ill person, one should do so in a manner different from that which one would adopt on an ordinary day of the week, so long as doing so does not delay or compromise in any way the patient's care. For example, one should switch on the electric light with the back of one's hand or finger.[72]

Bringing a Light That is Already On

4a. If there is a need for a light in the room of a dangerously ill person, and there is a portable source of light with a long enough cord on in another room, one should bring in that lamp (if they can keep it turned on), rather than turn on another light (unless there is an immediate need for light in which case it should be turned on right away).

This is because one should, to whatever extent possible, minimize the degree to which one violates Shabbat, and transferring the lamp from one room to another is an infringement of only the rabbinical prohibition against moving a *Muktzeh* object, whereas turning on a light may involve Torah prohibitions.[73]

4b. One should turn on a light in the patient's room and not bring a lamp from another room if the light emitted by the other lamp is not sufficient for one's purposes **or** time is pressing and any delay is liable to endanger the patient.[74]

4c. Where necessary, one may turn a light on for a dangerously ill patient even when there is a lamp already on in a neighboring area, if making the lamp available to the patient will cause the neighbor considerable hardship and inconvenience.

An example of this occurs when the neighbor is asleep and one would have to wake him or her.[75]

---

[70] Ibid.
[71] *Lev Avraham* 13:78. See previous page at the beginning of this section for further clarification.
[72] *Shemirat Shabbat Kehilchatah* 32:63; *Nishmat Avraham OH* 307:1 (4). See previous page for further clarification.
[73] Ibid., 32:65.
[74] Ibid.
[75] Ibid.

Minimizing the Number of Lights Turned On

5.   In order to minimize the amount of transgression, the effect achieved by any forbidden activity which must be performed should be limited (as much as possible) to only what is needed for the person who is dangerously ill.

- Therefore, if a) one switch will turn on only one bulb, whereas another will turn on more than one, and b) all that is required is the light of only one bulb, then one should operate the switch that turns on only one bulb.[76]

- Similarly, when there are two bulbs, one large and one small, that one could turn on for the purposes of a dangerously ill person, but either one of them alone would suffice to serve the patient's needs, it is better to turn on the smaller bulb in order not to ignite excess filament.[77]

Type of Light

6a.   Turning on an incandescent light bulb violates a Torah prohibition against creating a flame (see grey box on pg. 25). There was a time when fluorescent lights contained starters which produced a spark and heated up when turned on and were thus also considered a Torah prohibition, but since it was a smaller wire than those in an incandescent bulb, if one had to choose between the two, it was preferable to turn on a fluorescent bulb instead of an incandescent one.[78] However, most modern fluorescent lights (including screw-in compact fluorescents) have an electric ignition, not this starter or heating element, and are thus not biblically prohibited on Shabbat according to most opinions.

6b.   LCD, LED, and neon lights do not contain metal filaments and their use does not violate a Torah prohibition. When a light must be turned on for a dangerously ill person, such lights should thus be chosen if there is an option. For example, writing on a computer screen is preferred to writing with ink, and using a phone system with LED lights is better than using one with a bulb and light-up buttons.[79]

Using a Light Turned On for a Sick Person

7.   A light which was turned on during Shabbat for a person whose life is in danger may also be used by other people for any permitted reason since it was turned on in a permissible manner.[80]

Turning Off the Light

8a.   One may turn off a light on Shabbat to enable a dangerously ill person, for whom sleep is beneficial, to go to sleep, but one may do so only if it is not possible to safely cover, or move the light out of the room without extinguishing it.[81]

---

[76] Ibid., 32:66.
[77] Ibid., 32:67. This concern is primarily limited to incandescent bulbs, but since most hospitals use fluorescents, it is usually irrelevant. See the beginning of this section for further clarification.
[78] Ibid., 32:67 fn. 178.
[79] Rabbi Mechel Handler & Rabbi Dovid Weinberger, *Madrich L'chevra Hatzalah*, (Feldheim Publishers, 2008), 41-42.
[80] *Shemirat Shabbat Kehilchatah* 32:69.
[81] Another option is to reset a timer (which has been operating since before Shabbat) to turn off the light after a short interval.

8b. If the patient is incapacitated but not dangerously ill, a light may only be turned off for their sake if it is turned off in an abnormal manner, or by someone who is not Jewish, or if it is being turned off for multiple patients (at least three).[82]

If possible, one should turn the light off in a way which one would not use on a weekday, for instance by switching off the electricity with the back of one's hand, or asking someone who is not Jewish to do it [see **pg. 23-24**, for an explanation of these concepts].[83]

9. It is preferable to reduce the light through a dimmer, and not completely shut it off, if possible.[84]

Refrigerator Lights

10a. Before Shabbat, one should disconnect or remove the internal light of a refrigerator one is going to use on Shabbat, so as to prevent its being automatically turned on by the opening of the door.[85] Nevertheless, even if one has not done so, one may open the refrigerator on Shabbat (ideally in an abnormal manner) to remove whatever one needs for a patient whose life is in danger, despite the fact that this will cause the light inside to turn on. It would be preferable to ask someone who is not Jewish to open the door, if possible.[86]

10b. While the door is open, one may also make use of the opportunity to take out food for other people who are not dangerously ill.

10c. A Jew should not close the door of a refrigerator whose internal light will thereby be extinguished, unless all of the following conditions are met:

- There are still things in the refrigerator which are, or may possibly be, required on that Shabbat, or even after Shabbat, for a person whose life is in danger;

- The items one has in the refrigerator for the patient will spoil if the door is not closed;

- One will not be able to obtain other such items in their place;

- There is no other place where these items could be kept (e.g., in a neighbor's refrigerator).[87]

10d. It is permitted to ask someone who is not Jewish to open the refrigerator, even though the light will turn on, even for the needs of a person who is merely suffering from a minor ailment.[88]

---

[82] *Lev Avraham* 13:79 with clarification from Dr. Abraham via personal communication. See also *Shemirat Shabbat Kehilchatah* 33 fn. 25 for an explanation of why we are more stringent about turning off a light than other rabbinic prohibitions. These rulings may vary slightly based on the type of light being used. See grey box at the binging of this section.

[83] Ibid. 32:70; *Shulchan Aruch OH* 178:1, *Mishnah Berurah* 178:2; *Shulchan Aruch OH* 328:12 *Rema*.

[84] *Lev Avraham* 13:29.

[85] *Shemirat Shabbat Kehilchatah* 32:71.

[86] *Lev Avraham* 13:32; *Nishmat Avraham* OH 328:13 (1).

[87] *Shemirat Shabbat Kehilchatah* 32:71.

[88] *Igrot Moshe OH* 2:68.

11. In a case where one does close the refrigerator door, if they may have to open it again for the patient on that Shabbat, one should, before closing the door, disconnect or remove the internal bulb (and, if possible, one should do so in a manner one would not normally adopt). This will prevent the bulb from being turned on and off each time one has to open and close the door.[89]

Electric Warming Blankets

12. A patient who is dangerously ill may turn on an electric warming blanket if a regular blanket will not suffice (it should ideally be turned on by someone who is not Jewish, or if it must be done by a Jew it should be turned on in an abnormal manner).[90] It is also advisable to cover its electricity regulator as a reminder, so that no one will adjust the temperature unnecessarily.[91]

Heater and Air Conditioning

13a. Since cold is liable to harm a person who is dangerously ill, if the patient is cold and somebody who is not Jewish is unavailable, a Jew may turn a heater on for them if it warms the patient better than simply piling on additional blankets would do. When possible, one should vary their normal method of turning on the heater [see **pg. 23**, for an explanation of this concept].[92]

13b. If the heat becomes oppressive for a dangerously ill patient, one may turn it down. If this is insufficient and it is not possible to remove the heater from the room or easily transfer the patient to a cooler room, one may turn the heater off.[93]

14a. On a day when heat is oppressive and burdensome to a dangerously ill patient, if somebody who is not Jewish is unavailable, one may activate the air conditioning or a fan. If it becomes too cold, it may be turned off unless the air can be faced in a different direction or the patient may easily be transferred elsewhere.[94] In many circumstances the same may be true for a patient who is incapacitated but not dangerously ill (see grey box at the beginning of this section).

14b. For both the heater and air conditioner, when possible, one should vary their normal method of adjusting the temperature or turning off the mechanism. For example, one should use their elbows or wrists instead of their hands [see **pg. 23**, for an explanation of this concept].[95]

15. When the temperature is very uncomfortable, even if the patient is not dangerously ill, one may ask someone who is not Jewish to turn on the heat or air conditioning for them.[96]

---

[89] *Shemirat Shabbat Kehilchatah* 32:71.
[90] *Lev Avraham* 13:30. It is also advisable to cover its electricity regulator as a reminder, so that no one will adjust the temperature unnecessarily (Shemirat Shabbat Kehilchatah 38:7).
[91] *Shemirat Shabbat Kehilchatah* 38:7.
[92] Ibid., 32:83.
[93] Ibid., 32:85.
[94] Ibid., 32:86.
[95] Ibid.
[96] Ibid., 38:8-9. In many cases activating an air conditioner or a fan will not involve a Torah prohibition and may be permitted for a patient who is ill, even if not dangerously so, though it should be done in an abnormal manner. See further explanation on page 24.

E. Elevators, Electric Doors and Automatic Sensors on Shabbat

1a. Some authorities do not permit entering an elevator on Shabbat, even an automatic "Sabbath elevator," and even accompanying someone who is not Jewish (except to care for someone who is dangerously ill).[97]

1b. However, *Shemirat Shabbat Kehilchatah* states: "It is forbidden to use an elevator on Shabbat or *Yom Tov*, unless all of the following conditions are fulfilled:

1) The elevator operates automatically, that is to say it goes up and down by itself at fixed intervals or continuously;
2) The elevator stops by itself at the required floors, without the need for any human interference, whether by way of pressing buttons or otherwise;
3) The doors open and close automatically, likewise without the need for any human interference;
4) No prohibited act is involved in entering or leaving the elevator."[98]

There are, however, eminent authorities who allow the use of an elevator (subject to the above conditions) even for descending."[99]

2. The *Shemirat Shabbat Kehilchatah* continues, "one should not touch the electrically operated door of an elevator, either with one's hand or with one's body, when it is about to close."[100] One should be especially careful not to block the elevator doorway or interfere with these doors when they are closing. One should therefore enter and exit the elevator as soon as the door opens, or as others do so as well, so as not to affect the electric eye.[101]

3. The *Shemirat Shabbat Kehilchatah* continues, "There are some who permit the use of an elevator only for ascending, and not for descending [for reasons outlined in paragraph 4], even

a) When all the above conditions are fulfilled or
b) When the elevator is being operated by a non-Jew for their own purposes.

4. The *Shemirat Shabbat Kehilchatah* continues,

1. "The objections to descending in an elevator on Shabbat or *Yom Tov* stem from the way in which most modern elevators operate. The weight of the passengers can:

b) cause the elevator to descend more quickly and
c) affect the amount of current passing through the motor.[102]

---

[97] *Chelkat Yaakov* 3:137.
[98] *Shemirat Shabbat Kehilchatah* 23:49 (English edition), see 23:58 in Hebrew edition.
[99] Ibid.
[100] Ibid.
[101] *B'shvilei Beit Harefuah*, 20:5.
[102] This is based on the assumption that the weight of a passenger riding on an elevator assists the elevator's motor in the descent of the elevator, as Rav Levi Yitzchak Halperin, of the Institute for Science and Halacha in Jerusalem writes, "If the passenger is responsible for the descent, he is responsible also for illuminating the various lamps, connecting the door motor, the brakes, and numerous other electric circuits which are activated during the descent" (*Maaliot Bishabbat*, p. 11 of the English section). Furthermore, "When the car is descending with a heavy passenger load it may speed up to a point where the counter-force developed in the motor is greater than the force of the electric

2. It is argued that a Torah prohibition (and not just a rabbinical restriction) is involved when lights are turned on or powered as a result of these factors.[103]

3. This is of course disputed by the eminent authorities who permit the use of an elevator for descending (subject to the conditions set out in the previous paragraphs)."[104]

5. The English edition of the *Shemirat Shabbat Kehilchatah* notes that, "Due to the complicated technicalities involved and the differences of opinion among the authorities, one would be well advised not to use an elevator on Shabbat or *Yom Tov* without consulting a properly qualified rabbi."[105] That said, it should be noted that, "although many Orthodox Jews do not use automatic elevators at all, they are technically permitted."[106] As Rav Shlomo Zalman Auerbach concludes, "It is permitted to ride in a descending elevator [in addition to an ascending elevator] even if it is not a case of loss… so one should not rebuke those who are lenient and ride on a descending automatic elevator."[107]

6. One who is dangerously ill may be transported in a regular elevator on Shabbat, and a healthy person may even accompany them, if they are needed. They may also push the buttons to summon the elevator for the dangerously ill patient, even if it causes a light to illuminate, though it should be pressed in an abnormal manner.[108]

7. A Jew may not, however, summon an elevator for a patient who is not dangerously ill, though one may ask someone who is not Jewish to summon the elevator by pushing the buttons if the patient needs to be transported for the sake of their treatment.[109]

8. A visitor who must use an elevator, and is unable to use an automatic "Sabbath elevator," should ideally let someone who is not Jewish press the button to summon the elevator or select the floor level (though the same concerns regarding descending, affecting the doors, etc., would be relevant in such a case as well).[110] They should either hint at which floor they need pressed, hoping someone who is not Jewish will press the button for them, or they must simply exit at the closest floor to their destination and take the stairs, if possible.

9. If no one is around to assist, <u>in a case of great need</u>, one may press the button themselves in an unusual manner, i.e., using their knuckles or two hands.[111]

---

power station. When this condition occurs, the motor, rather than aiding the descent, is used to brake the car thus preventing dangerous over speeding. When the speed of a motor increases to a value above that for which it was designed, it automatically becomes a generator. Instead of consuming electrical energy it generates power which is fed into the electric company lines to be used by consumers in the immediate vicinity" (*Maaliot Bishabbat*, p. 19 of the English section).

[103] It should be noted, however, that today most lights that are turned on are not Torah prohibitions.

[104] *Shemirat Shabbat Kehilchatah* 23:50 (English edition), see 23:58 in the Hebrew edition and footnotes 164 & 166 for Rav Shlomo Zalman Auerbach's detailed explanation of why entering such an elevator is permitted.

[105] Ibid., 23:49, (English edition vol. 2 pg. 342).

[106] *Shemirat Shabbat Kehilchatah* 23:58.

[107] Ibid., 23 fn. 166.

[108] *Lev Avraham* 13:130; *Nishmat Avraham* OH 307:1 (4).

[109] Ibid., 13:131. There may be room for more leniency depending on the type of electricity involved. See grey box on page 24.

[110] *Shemirat Shabbat Kehilchatah* 23:59.

[111] *Madrich L'chevra Hatzalah*, 144.

10. The *Shemirat Shabbat Kehilchatah* writes, "One may use automatic escalators and moving sidewalks that operate continuously."[112]

11a. One should always attempt to use only the manually opened doors, rather than automatic electric eye doors, as the *Shemirat Shabbat Kehilchatah* writes, "It is prohibited, both on Shabbat and *Yom Tov*, to pass through an electrically operated automatic door which is opened by means of a photo-electric cell or when one treads on the floor in front of it. In both of these cases, by approaching the door, one would be activating an electrical current."[113]

11b. If one is in an area where their only choice is to use an automatic door and one needs to enter for the sake of a patient, one should:

- ideally enter together at the same time as someone who is not Jewish, if that is not possible, one may

- ask someone who is not Jewish to open the doors for them. If neither of these are possible, another option is to

- ask someone who does not know that their entering will cause the door to open, so that it will be considered "*Mitasek*" (when a person intends to do a permitted act, and accidentally does a prohibited act).[114]

11c. If none of these options are possible, such as in the middle of the night, one may cause the door to open in an abnormal manner, such as by extending one's foot or arm instead of one's entire body.[115]

12. It is permitted to pass in front of a closed circuit video camera on Shabbat, such as a security camera, because the video is only recorded temporarily (and it is thus not considered permanent writing) and it is not intended even though it is a "*Psik Reisha*" (an inevitable consequence).[116]

13. Water faucets that flow automatically when triggered by an electric sensor that recognizes hands placed beneath them may not be used on Shabbat unless it is a case of danger to the patient.[117] One must use a hand sanitizer or find a manually operated faucet on Shabbat.

14. Restrooms that are equipped with lights that automatically illuminate and function when a person enters, and turn off when a person exits, should not be used on Shabbat. However, in a case of great need, if it is impossible to find an alternative restroom, one may use such a restroom on Shabbat.[118] If possible, one should insure that there is a light that remains on in the room throughout Shabbat or if this is not

---

[112] *Shemirat Shabbat Kehilchatah* 23:52.

[113] Ibid., 23:53.

[114] *Chasdei Avraham*, vol. 2, pg. 197 (with clarification from the author in personal communication). Another option is to allow a child, even if he or she is Jewish, to open the door—ideally in an abnormal manner.

[115] Ibid., 198; See also *Lev Avraham* 13:132, who permits passing through an electric door in the normal manner if there is no other option and the need is great.

[116] *Lev Avraham* 13:139; Rav Moshe Feinstein, in *Techumim* vol. 14, 433.

[117] *B'Shvilei Beit Harefuah*, 20:8.

[118] Ibid., 20:9. This is based on the great need of this particular situation and human dignity considerations of one who must use the restroom, coupled with the possibility that causing a light to turn on via an electric eye is not the normal manner of turning on a light.

possible, leave the door slightly ajar so that they are not getting benefit solely from the light that was initiated by their action on Shabbat.[119]

15.	There are often places in a hospital where automatic functions, such as doors, are neutralized but the electric sensor is still functioning (i.e., it may blink or otherwise register one's motion, but does not result in an action, such as opening a door or turning on a light). A person may nevertheless go through an area that may trigger such a sensor, particularly if they don't know that it is taking place.[120]

F. The Use of a Telephone

1.	The *Shemirat Shabbat Kehilchatah* writes: "When one has to telephone a doctor to come, or for instructions as to treatment, one should, where possible, remove the receiver in a manner which differs from that which one would use on an ordinary day of the week. For instance, one should displace the receiver with one's elbow or wrist, or in the event that this is not possible, one should lift it off its rest together with another person, or if nobody else is there, one should take it off with both hands at the same time."[121]

2a.	"At the end of the conversation, one should not replace the receiver on its rest, except in the following circumstances, when it *must* be replaced:

	1)	If one may need to take an incoming call that Shabbat on the same instrument or line for the purpose of saving human life.
	2)	If there is reason to suppose the number one has called may be needed again that Shabbat in connection with saving human life."[122]

2b.	A cell phone call should be made, and concluded, by pressing the buttons in an abnormal manner, such as with the back of ones fingers, when possible.[123]

3.	A cordless telephone should not be returned to its base, which would cause its battery to be charged, unless that phone may be needed again on Shabbat for life-saving purposes and, if it were not returned to its base, it would not be usable again that Shabbat.[124]

4.	"When speaking on the telephone for the purposes of a dangerously ill patient, one is not obligated to be sparing in words, weighing each word to see whether it is required, but one should say everything that has to be said concerning the patient. One may even end the conversation with some such phrases as, 'Goodbye,' or 'Thank you very much.' However, one should certainly not talk about matters which have no connection with the patient or their treatment."[125]

---

[119]	Ibid. By doing this, the action falls into the category of a "*Psik Reisha D'lo Nicha Lei*" (an inevitable consequence that one does not need).

[120]	Ibid., 20:7.

[121]	*Shemirat Shabbat Kehilchatah* 32:40.

[122]	Ibid., 32:42. One should ideally replace the receiver onto the base in an unusual manner, such as with two hands (ibid., 32:40 & *Nishmat Avraham OH* 338:1).

[123]	*Nishmat Avraham OH* 338:1

[124]	Ibid., 32:41. In such a case one should put the receiver back on its rest in an abnormal manner (34:42).

[125]	Ibid., 32:41.

What type of phone to use

5. Because one must always try to select the lesser violation in non-life-threatening situations and attempt to minimize the extent and severity of Shabbat transgression, if one has to use an electrical device, they should choose one that does not produce light or heat.[126]

6. Although it was once considered completely forbidden to use a telephone for the sake of a non-seriously ill patient, since most phones today use neon or LED lights which are not considered "fire,"[127] one may use a telephone for a patient with a non-life-threatening illness when necessary, though it should be done in an abnormal manner.[128]

Informing others of the situation in the hospital by phone

7a. One should call the family of a patient who is dangerously ill if the patient arrives at the hospital unconscious on Shabbat and in need of someone to direct their care and ensure that they have the appropriate doctors, treatment and guidance.[129] If the patient is lonely or has some other concern that they would like to notify others about via telephone, a call may not be made unless it can reasonably be seen as a life-saving matter (or preventing the patient's condition from deteriorating into a life-threatening condition).[130]

7b. A patient (or their visitor) may ask someone who is not Jewish to call someone if the patient's situation is very poor and declining on Shabbat. If there is a great need for them to assist or be with the patient, and the patient indicates that they need this person to be with them, they may be driven to the hospital by someone who is not Jewish if this can help improve the patient's condition. If this is not possible, and one is needed to assist a dangerously ill patient, share medical information with the staff, or even just to be by the bedside of the dangerously ill patient to provide support and encourage the staff to take the best care of the patient, a Jew may even drive him or herself to the hospital on Shabbat.[131]

7c. The phone may not be used for a non-critical situation, such as to inform family members of the gender of a child born on Shabbat or to inform family members of a death.

7d. However, if it will alleviate the patient's anxiety, one may have a staff member who is not Jewish call someone if they have a person who is not Jewish available to answer the phone, or an answering machine, to inform them of the patient's medical status.[132]

---

[126] When using a cell phone, one should also open the mouthpiece and dial the numbers in an abnormal fashion if doing so would not delay urgent patient care (*Lev Avraham,* 13:49).

[127] This is because these lights do not contain a filament that glows.

[128] *Lev Avraham* 13:84; *Nishmat Avraham OH* 278 fn. 139.

[129] *Shevet Halevi* 8:65.

[130] Ibid. It should be noted that being terrified is often considered life-threatening "*Pikuach Nefesh.*"

[131] *Chasdei Avraham,* vol. 2, 237-240; *Nishmat Avraham OH* 278:1 (29), pg. 236.

[132] Rabbi Dovid Weinberger, *Guide for the Jewish Hospital Patient,* Orthodox Union, 24 (On pg. 36 he writes in the name of Rav Shlomo Zalman Auerbach that if one's family does not have someone who is not Jewish available to answer or an answering machine, then they may have a non-Jew call their family and leave a message via a specific pre-arranged symbol, such as one or two rings, to inform them of the birth and gender of the child if this will alleviate the patient's anxiety).

G. Use of the Call Button & Adjustable Bed

1.   One who is ill, even if not dangerously so [see **pg. 16**, for an explanation of this concept], and needs their nurse does not have to wait until the nurse checks in on them but may push the call button in an unusual manner, (such as with the back of their finger).[133]

2.   Similarly, if necessary, a patient who is very uncomfortable may adjust their mechanical bed on their own, in an unusual manner, if there is nobody available to do it for them.[134]

H. Parking and Turning off a Car[135]

1.   *Shemirat Shabbat Kehilchatah* states, "A driver who has brought a dangerously ill patient to the hospital should leave their car parked at the spot where it has come to a halt at the end of the journey, unless it could be a potential source of danger in that position. They must not drive the car further than is essential for the welfare of the patient, merely in order to avoid the risk of being fined for parking in a forbidden area."[136]

2.   "If the engine is still operating after one has come to a halt, one may ask someone who is not Jewish to turn it off (but it is better to just tell him that the engine is still on and let him draw his own conclusion as to what he ought to do). If there is no one who is not Jewish available, then, subject to the contents of the next paragraph, there is room for taking a lenient attitude and

1) Having the engine switched off by a boy under age thirteen or a girl under twelve, or
2) In the absence of a minor, turning the engine off oneself, preferably in an unusual manner."[137]

3.   Although one should not switch off the engine if it will cause any lights to illuminate or turn off since this is not part of the effort to save the patient's life,[138] "An exception occurs, and one may have the engine turned off by a minor or even turn it off oneself (if no one who is not Jewish is available), when leaving the car with the engine running would create public danger, as where

---

[133] Rabbi Gershon Bess, based on *Mishnah Berurah* 328:57. If the patient is dangerously ill they do not even need to push the button in an unusual manner. See also *Nishmat Avraham OH* 338:1 & *Shemirat Shabbat Kehilchatah* 40:23.

[134] Ibid.

[135] Because this guide is intended to assist people who face challenges pertaining to Jewish Law in a hospital setting, all of the complicated rulings related to driving cars on Shabbat in an emergency situation are beyond the scope of this work (see *Shemirat Shabbat Kehilchatah* 40:60-86 for that discussion). We will instead limit ourselves to the issues that take place at the hospital itself.

[136] *Shemirat Shabbat Kehilchatah* 40:57. One should thus not leave the car right in front of the hospital entrance, where it could obstruct the access of the other drivers bringing emergency cases for treatment. One should thus stop before actually reaching the hospital entrance, or drive sufficient distance beyond the entrance to avoid interfering with the traffic to the hospital.

[137] Ibid., 40:59.

[138] Ibid., 40:60.

1) There is reasonable fear that the continuous running of the engine will make it overheat, causing the radiator to explode and injure passersby, or

2) There is a risk of children playing with the car."[139]

4. However, this is usually permitted since a vehicle may be needed again for a seriously ill patient and leaving the headlights on for the patient's needs. The exception is when the vehicle will be needed again for a seriously ill patient and leaving the headlights on may result in difficulty restarting the car.[140]

5. The ignition keys should be left in the car since they are *Muktzeh* (an object one is forbidden to carry on Shabbat).[141] However, if they are also used for opening the car's doors[142] or if other keys, such as one's house keys, are also on the key chain, one may carry all of the keys together.[143] Furthermore, if there is a real possibility that the car would get stolen if the ignition key is left in it, it may be removed.[144]

6. If there are people who are not Jewish available to park one's car for them [see **pg. 24**, for an explanation of this concept], they should be asked to do so rather than turning the car off oneself.[145] Ideally this should be done simply by hinting to the fact that it would be appreciated if the person who is not Jewish did this on one's behalf, rather than directly asking them to do so.[146]

7. If upon exiting the car a light will go on, the light should be turned off first so that it will not light up when the door is opened. If lights will still turn on, the door should be opened and closed in an abnormal manner, such as using the back of one's hand, or two hands to open it, or closing it with their elbow or foot.[147]

I. Discharge on Shabbat/Holidays

Driving Home from the Hospital on Shabbat/Use of a Taxi

1a. A doctor, ambulance driver, or any other person who has driven where needed for the sake of a dangerously ill patient is not allowed to drive a car back on Shabbat except in the following circumstances:

1) They are required to make another trip for a person whose life may be in danger, or

2) There is a reasonable likelihood that they will be required to make another such journey (e.g., the doctor is "on call" and may be contacted later on Shabbat to care for a different patient in some other location).[148]

---

[139] Ibid.
[140] Ibid., 40:69.
[141] Ibid., 20:80.
[142] Ibid.
[143] Ibid., 20:86 fn. 309.
[144] *Lev Avraham*, 13:55.
[145] *B'shvilei Beit Harafuah, Dinei Shabbat*, 9:1.
[146] *Shemirat Shabbat Kehilchatah*, 40 fn. 151.
[147] *Madrich L'chevra Hatzalah*, 118.
[148] *Shemirat Shabbat Kehilchatah* 40:79-81. *Lev Avraham* 13, fn. 188 points out that since doctors have cell phones today, there is often less of a pressing need for them to return home on Shabbat to be available near their telephones.

1b. A doctor may return home with a non-Jewish driver [see **pg. 24**, for an explanation of this concept], and may even call a taxi to take them to the hospital instead of driving oneself (assuming the delay does not endanger the patient) so that the taxi will be available to drive the doctor back home afterwards.[149]

1c. Even when one may drive back, the driver may not:

1) Stop on the way or make a detour from the shortest route back to their base, except for reasons connected with the saving of human life, nor

2) When one reaches their destination, they may not travel farther than is essential to enable them to fulfill their duties in the event of another call.[150]

2a. A patient who is discharged on Shabbat and has nowhere to go, or a visitor who must return home (such as parents who are needed to tend to their children), and for whom it is difficult to remain in the hospital over Shabbat should not return home with a Jewish driver, even if the driver him or herself is allowed to drive (such as a doctor or ambulance driver as mentioned above).[151] Instead, one should ask someone who is not Jewish to call a car service to bring them home.[152] If there is no one else to call the taxi, it is preferable to call it oneself rather than to drive a car on Shabbat, since making a phone call is one rabbinic prohibition and driving a car on Shabbat involves constant Biblical transgressions of "kindling" every moment that the car is driving.[153]

2b. If one has permission to travel in a car operated by someone who is not Jewish, it is ideal if they can arrange with the driver to pay the fare after Shabbat, even if this means that they will have to promise the driver a better tip, as it is preferable to paying on Shabbat. Another option is to request that someone who is not Jewish pay the driver for them. If this cannot be worked out, one can use a prepaid ticket, or if this is not possible, one may even take money with them and pay the fare on Shabbat, but should not accept change from the driver. One should ideally show the driver where the money is so that he can remove it himself and one will not be forced to handle money on Shabbat, but if the driver does not agree, then one can hand the driver the money directly. Nevertheless, this should ideally be done only after consultation with a rabbinic authority, as it may lead others to conclude that one is violating Shabbat without justification.[154]

3. If one is leaving the hospital on Shabbat and has in their possession valuable *Muktzeh* objects, or if there is not a local reliable *Eruv*, and if there is no place where they can securely leave their possessions in the hospital until after Shabbat, they should be taken with them in an irregular manner,[155] such as placing the objects inside one's shoes or between the clothes that they are wearing. One should not keep them in their hand or pocket unless they are needed for the safety of a patient.[156]

---

[149] Ibid., 40:81. The *Shemirat Shabbat Kehilchatah* points out that a doctor may call a taxi to return home with a non-Jewish driver even if there is no pressing need, but the doctor prefers to be at home. See also *Nishmat Avraham OH* 329:9 (3) & 278:4 (46).

[150] Ibid., 40:79.

[151] *Madrich L'chevra Hatzalah*, 114-115.

[152] *Shemirat Shabbat Kehilchatah*, 40:81. The taxi driver cannot be Jewish.

[153] Ibid., 40 fn. 176.

[154] *Shemirat Shabbat Kehilchatah* 38:13, *Lev Avraham* 13:68.

[155] *Nishmat Avraham OH* 252:7 (5).

[156] *Shemirat Shabbat Kehilchata* 32:54.

J. Writing on Shabbat

1. Writing on Shabbat is a Torah prohibition which includes writing any meaningful symbols.[157] Therefore, one who arrives at the hospital on Shabbat may not sign in upon admittance or check off boxes on a form. However, they may tell all of their necessary information to someone who is not Jewish [see **pg. 24**, for an explanation of this concept], even if it will result in that person writing the information down.[158]

2. If a patient is asked to sign a consent for the performance of an urgent procedure or treatment, they should explain that they cannot sign it on Shabbat and instead give verbal consent before witnesses. If the hospital management is not satisfied with this, one may sign a document if:

    a) The patient's life is, or may be, in danger **and**

    b) The hospital management makes the performance of the operation conditional on the prior consent of the patient or their relatives.[159] (The method of signing is described below in 3c & 3d.)

3a. *Shemirat Shabbat Kehilchatah* states: "A Jewish doctor may write anything which has to be written on Shabbat for a person whose life is in danger. This could include, by way of example,

    a) Urgent prescriptions for medicines,

    b) An urgent letter referring a patient to a hospital, and

    c) Important medical particulars which are liable to be forgotten, or confused with those of another patient, if left unrecorded.

3b. However, it is forbidden to write down something which does not directly affect the patient's treatment (for instance, that he belongs to a medical insurance plan).

3c. Moreover, one must limit oneself to writing the absolute minimum without which one would be unable to do what is necessary to save the patient, and one must not add even one more letter than needed, or a period at the end of the sentence.[160]

3d. One should try to write whatever is essential in a manner different from that which one would adopt another day of the week, for example by using one's left hand.[161] Of course, where speed is vital and writing in a different manner is liable to result in delay, one should write in one's usual way."[162]

4. Because one should always attempt to do the fewest possible transgressions, if one must write and they have a choice, it is preferable to write on a computer which has already been turned on than to write on paper by hand.[163]

---

[157] *Mishnah Berurah* 306:47. See also *Nishmat Avraham OH* 340:4 (6) for a detailed summary and discussion of these rules.

[158] *Chasdei Avraham* vol. 2, 15:3.

[159] *Shemirat Shabbat Kehilchatah* 40:25.

[160] Ibid., 32:48.

[161] It should be noted that although using one's weaker hand is considered "abnormal" enough with regards to writing, it is not always considered sufficiently abnormal to permit other prohibited actions. For example, carrying where there is no *Eruv*, turning on a switch, lifting a telephone handset, writing on a computer, or erasing would all have to be done in a more "abnormal manner" than using one's weaker hand, such as using one's elbow or back of the hand. See *Mishnah Berurah* 340:22 (end); *B'Shvilei Beit Harefuah*, 7.

[162] *Shemirat Shabbat Kehilchatah* 32:49.

[163] *Shulchan Shlomo Hilchot Shabbat* 340:4 (11); *Shemirat Shabbat Kehilchatah* 32:48; *Nishmat Avraham OH*

5. A patient who is on a respirator and has no method of communication other than writing things that cannot be hinted may write whatever is needed. If possible however, this patient should still attempt to write with their non-writing hand, and use as few words and letters as possible to get the message across.[164]

6a. The *Shemirat Shabbat Kehilchatah* writes: "When a patient is discharged from the hospital on Shabbat, it is forbidden to write out, or to request a Jew to write out, a certificate of discharge on Shabbat.

6b. One may ask someone who is not Jewish to write out the certificate, if:

1) The patient is still ill, even though not dangerously so.
2) The patient needs further treatment, as specified in the certificate, **and**
3) It will not be possible to obtain the certificate after Shabbat, or waiting will cause a delay in the treatment."[165]

6c. If one is in a situation where their refusal to leave their room would cause pain to another person who needs the space, it is permitted to ask someone who is not Jewish to sign the forms for them so that the patient can be discharged, even if he or she is now fully healthy.[166]

7. A patient who chooses to discharge themselves from the hospital against their physician's recommendation is not permitted to sign a form, such as a release of liability, nor may they ask someone who is not Jewish to sign it for them. Rather, one should gather two witnesses (such as nurses) who can testify that the patient understands the decision that they are making, and this may be written down after Shabbat ends.[167]

K. Shabbat Candles

> Every Friday before sundown, traditionally observant Jews light candles to usher in the Sabbath, thereby fulfilling an obligation designed to provide an atmosphere of tranquility and increase the honor and joy of the day. Lighting candles for holidays is discussed in the section on Festivals.

LIGHTING AN ACTUAL FLAME INSIDE THE HOSPITAL IS VERY DANGEROUS AND FORBIDDEN; THEREFORE "CANDLES" IN THIS SECTION REFER TO ELECTRIC LIGHTS, AS WILL BE DISUCSSED BELOW.

1a. One who is not married should light Shabbat and festival candles even when they are in the hospital. One who is married may have their husband or wife light candles at home and say the blessing, which releases them from the obligation to light candles themselves.[168]

340:4(6:11 & 22). Printing out what has been written on the computer is a Torah prohibition, and should thus not be done by someone who is Jewish unless it is absolutely essential for a dangerously ill patient and there is nobody else available to do it for them, in which case it should be done in an abnormal manner such as by pressing the buttons with the back of one's hand (*Nishmat Avraham OH* 340:4 (6:11 s.v."Hadfasa")).

[164] *Nishmat Avraham OH* 328:Intro 6(5).
[165] *Shemirat Shabbat Kehilchatah* 40:44 (40:54 in Hebrew edition).
[166] *Lev Avraham* 13:118.
[167] Ibid., 13:120.
[168] *Shemirat Shabbat Kehilchatah* 45:6.

1b. Nonetheless, it is customary for a traditionally observant married Jewish woman to light her own candles and to recite the blessing, if she wishes, even if there is someone to light candles in her home.[169]

1c. A man who prefers to have his wife fulfill his obligation by lighting candles at home, should still have candles lit in honor of Shabbat in his room, but should do so without reciting the blessing, as long as there is other light in the room.[170]

2. One who is able to get out of bed should light the candles near the table at which they will eat. If not, someone else should light them on the patient's behalf, or the patient should light them near their bedside, where they will eat, and the candles should ideally not be removed.[171]

3a. One is not permitted to light a fire in a hospital. Therefore, one's only option for lighting Shabbat and festival candles is to use electric lights. The *Shemirat Shabbat Kehilchatah* writes, "There are authorities who hold that the *Mitzvah* can be satisfactorily performed by turning on electric light bulbs. A person who does this should recite the appropriate blessing in the usual way, provided they indeed switch on the lights in honor of Shabbat."[172] However, a blessing should not be recited on electric Shabbat candles that do not provide any illumination to the room.

3b. Some say that it is best to simply turn on the regular lights, since they illuminate the room well, in honor of Shabbat and to recite the blessing on them instead of on small candles or a flashlight.[173]

3c. If one is lighting electric candles, it may be ideal to use battery-operated candles, such as a flashlight, in which there is sufficient energy to insure that the lights will remain lit at least until the time one begins their nighttime Shabbat meal.[174]

4. A blessing should not be made on lighting candles which will not be able to be enjoyed by oneself or anyone else on Shabbat, as this would be a blessing made unnecessarily.[175] Therefore, one who will be taken from their room into a procedure before Shabbat begins and is not likely to regain consciousness until it is impossible to benefit from the lit candles on Shabbat, should not light the candles with a blessing.[176]

5. Although one may make use of the illumination provided by Shabbat lights for any purpose, one should not do anything in the glow of their lights which shows

---

[169] Ibid., 45:6.

[170] *B'shvilei Beit Harefuah*, Shabbat 3:9.

[171] Ibid., 36:16; *B'shvilei Beit Harefuah*, Shabbat 3:8.

[172] *Shemirat Shabbat Kehilchatah* 43:4. According to most authorities, the illumination for Shabbat candles can be provided by either incandescent or fluorescent light. To make it clear that one is turning the lights on in honor of Shabbat they should turn off the other lights in the room before turning on the Shabbat candles and then turn the lights that they will need over Shabbat back on in honor of Shabbat, and one must make sure not to turn on their candles before "*Plag Haminchah*" (1¼ halachic hours before sunset). See *Shulchan Aruch OH* 263:4.

[173] *B'shvilei Beit Harefuah*, Shabbat 3:6. Others rule that one should use special electric Shabbat candles which are designed to make it clear that their purpose is to honor Shabbat (*Tzitz Eliezer* 1:20:11).

[174] *Lev Avraham* 14:9; *Shemirat Shabbat Kehilchatah* 43 fn. 100. Other authorities disagree with this requirement, and permit lighting electric candles that are not battery-operated, see: *Yabia Omer OH* 2:17 and a related discussion in *Tzitz Eliezer* 1:20:12:2.

[175] *Mishnah Berurah* 263:30.

[176] *Nishmat Avraham OH* 263:4. The *Tzitz Eliezer* 15:32(6) however, does permit lighting candles with a blessing in such circumstances.

disrespect for the *Mitzvah* of Shabbat lights.[177] For example, a bedpan should not be used in the presence of Shabbat candles unless the patient is covered with a sheet.[178]

6. Although a woman who forgets to light Shabbat candles would ordinarily begin lighting one more candle on every subsequent Shabbat than had been her custom to light until then, if her failure to light candles was the result of illness (either her own illness or that of a family member whom she was tending to), she is not required to add a candle thereafter.[179]

L. *Kiddush & Havdalah*

The Torah commands us to verbally sanctify the Sabbath, "Remember the Sabbath day to make it holy" (Exodus 20:8). This means that one must single out this day and elevate it above the rest of the week with words of sanctity and praise.

To facilitate observance of this commandment, we recite the text of *"Kiddush"* (Sanctification) over a beverage (detailed below) prior to the evening and morning Sabbath meals.

1a. Once Shabbat has begun, both men and women[180] may not eat or drink anything, even water, until they recite or hear *Kiddush*.[181] However, one who is under doctor's orders to take medicine before their meals may take it prior to *Kiddush* and may also drink a little water (but no other drink) to help them swallow, if necessary.[182]

1b. One who is being fed through a tube, such as an IV, an NG tube, or a PEG, does not need to recite or hear *Kiddush* prior to being fed.[183] However, if one is able to hear someone else recite *Kiddush*, or if they can recite just the *"Vayechulu"* paragraph, it is a good practice.[184]

2. *Kiddush* should be recited using a nice, respectable cup in order to beautify the *Mitzvah*. One should therefore only use a disposable cup if they have no other option.[185] If one doesn't even have a disposable cup they may simply make Kiddush on the wine in the bottle (unless one has already drunk from that bottle).[186]

---

[177] *Shemirat Shabbat Kehilchatah* 43:41.
[178] *Lev Avraham* 14:3.
[179] *Shulchan Aruch OH* 263:1 *Rema; Mishnah Berurah* 263:7; *Shemirat Shabbat Kehilchatah* 43:3.
[180] *Shulchan Aruch OH* 271:2.
[181] Ibid., 271:4.
[182] *Shemirat Shabbat Kehilchatah* 52:3. This is because one is not intending to enjoy the water.
[183] *Minchat Yitzchak* 8:30; *Lev Avraham* 14:31 points out that they do not need to make blessings before and after being fed in this manner either.
[184] *Lev Avraham*, 14:31.
[185] *Igrot Moshe OH* 3:39 (However, the *Tzitz Eliezer* 12:23 writes that a disposable cup is perfectly permissible); *Shemirat Shabbat Kehilchatah* 47:11; *Shulchan Shlomo, Hilchot Shabbat* 271:18.
[186] *Shemirat Shabbat Kehilchatah* 47:11 & fn. 52.

What to recite *Kiddush* over

3a.   One should ideally recite *Kiddush* on wine or grape juice.[187] However, if one is unable to obtain wine or grape juice, or is unable to drink them, for the evening *Kiddush* they should not use another beverage, but should make *Kiddush* over two whole loaves of bread (or bread rolls).[188] If these are unavailable, then *Kiddush* may also be recited over a single slice of bread.[189] If even this is not available, one may recite *Kiddush* over cake or cookies made from wheat, barley, rye, oats or spelt.[190] If none of the above is available, one may recite *Kiddush* over an important drink,[191] detailed in paragraph 3c below.

* The order of priorities for Friday night would thus ideally be wine or grape juice; the next best would be bread or bread products; and lastly, an important drink other than wine.[192]

3b.   When making *Kiddush* over bread, the procedure is as follows:

- One should first wash their hands and say the blessing of *"Al Netilat Yadayim."*
- Then they recite *Kiddush* in the normal manner from the beginning, covering and holding the bread.
- When one concludes the *"Vayechulu"* paragraph, they uncover the bread and simply say the full blessing of *"Hamotzi Lechem Min Haaretz"* instead of *"Borei P'ri Hagafen."*
- One then finishes reciting the rest of *Kiddush* with the bread covered again and then eats the bread at the point where they would normally drink the wine.[193]

3c.   On Shabbat morning, if one is unable to use wine or grape juice, there is greater leniency regarding other accepted beverages.[194] Therefore, instead of reciting *Kiddush* over bread, one may recite *Kiddush* on a drink of consequence that is not normally consumed only to quench thirst, but would be served in honor of the meal and guests,[195] such as natural fruit juice or beer.[196] If this is not available, one may even recite *Kiddush* Shabbat morning over a cup of milk, coffee or sweetened tea.[197] One should not recite *Kiddush* over water, so if nothing else is available, *Kiddush* may be recited over bread Shabbat morning as well.[198]

* The order of priorities for Shabbat morning is thus ideally wine or grape juice; the next best would be an important drink other than wine; and lastly bread or bread products.[199]

---

[187]   *Shulchan Aruch OH* 272:2; *Minchat Shlomo* 1:4.

[188]   Ibid., 272:9.

[189]   *Mishnah Berurah* 274:2.

[190]   *Shemirat Shabbat Kehilchatah* 53:7. In such a case one should ideally eat enough of the cake or cookies to form a meal (i.e. the same as the amount of bread they would normally eat at a meal) and then wash their hands and recite the same *"Hamotzi"* and *"Birkat Hamazon"* blessings over them as they would over bread. If they do not have enough to do this, then they would simply recite the appropriate blessing for that food item, such as *"Mezonot"* (*Shemirat Shabbat Kehilchatah* 53:18; *Lev Avraham* 14:24).

[191]   *Lev Avraham* 14:23. However, the *Lev Avraham* points out that the *Sephardi* authorities rule that on Friday night one may not use anything other than wine or bread for *Kiddush.*

[192]   *Shemirat Shabbat Kehilchatah* 53 fn. 24.

[193]   Ibid., 53:15.

[194]   *Shulchan Aruch OH* 289:2

[195]   *Igrot Moshe OH* 2:75.

[196]   *Shemirat Shabbat Kehilchatah* 53:9. See also paragraph 8 below.

[197]   Ibid., 53:11.

[198]   Ibid., 53:12.

[199]   Ibid., 53 fn. 34.

One who is unable to recite *Kiddush*

4. One who was unable to recite *Kiddush* on Friday night, but is able to do so Shabbat morning, should recite the Friday evening *Kiddush* on Shabbat morning but omit the "*Vayechulu*" passage.[200]

5a. A patient who is unable to consume wine, grape juice, or bread, is exempt from reciting *Kiddush*. In such a case, one should ideally hear someone else recite *Kiddush*.[201] If this is not possible, then when one says the *Amidah* prayer they should have the intention during the benediction "*Mikadesh HaShabbat*" to include the *Mitzvah* of *Kiddush*, and would then be able to eat without making the usual *Kiddush*.[202] One who is simply unable to fulfill the *Mitzvah* of saying or hearing *Kiddush* should still fulfill the *Mitzvah* of eating their Shabbat meal, even without *Kiddush*.[203]

5b. If suitable beverages or bread become available later during the course of Shabbat, they should then be used to recite *Kiddush*.[204]

5c. Even if one knows that a suitable beverage or bread will be arriving later, they should not wait for them if they are weak and find it difficult to wait.[205]

6a. One who is feeling weak and must eat on Shabbat before saying the morning prayers should still recite *Kiddush* before eating, if they can. He should preferably first say at least the "*Birchot HaTorah*" blessings and the first paragraph of the *Shema* before reciting *Kiddush*.[206]

6b. However, one who is weak may eat as much as they need to strengthen themselves before praying or reciting Kiddush.[207]

Havdalah

As part of the commandment to honor the Sabbath, Jewish law requires one to make a verbal expression of its sanctity and holiness separate from the rest of the week at its conclusion with a service called "*Havdalah*" or "Distinction."

7a. Once Shabbat is over, one may not begin to do "work" until they have either said the "*Havdalah*" benediction during the *Amidah* prayer or recited the phrase "*Baruch Hamavdil Bein Kodesh L'chol*."[208]

7b. One may not partake of food or drink, other than water, until they have recited (or heard) the full *Havdalah* over wine (or other accepted beverage mentioned in the

---

[200] *Shulchan Aruch OH* 271:8; *Shemirat Shabbat Kehilchatah* 40:57. This is true even if they did fulfill the *Mitzvah* of *Kiddush* Friday night through having it in mind during the *Amidah* prayer (*Lev Avraham* 14:30).

[201] *Shulchan Aruch OH* 272:9 *Rema*.

[202] *Mishnah Berurah* 289:10; *Shemirat Shabbat Kehilchatah* 40:57.

[203] *Shemirat Shabbat Kehilchatah* 53:14.

[204] Ibid., 52:25.

[205] Ibid., 52:23.

[206] Ibid., 40:5. If it is difficult to say both the morning blessings and the "*Shema*" before eating, one can just say the "*Shema*" (*Mishnah Berurah* 99:22).

[207] *Mishnah Berurah* 286:9. See also *Shaar Hatziyun* 9 that one may certainly eat if necessary before *Mussaf*.

[208] *Shulchan Aruch OH* 299:10.

next paragraph).[209] However, someone who is weak may eat if they need food and are not yet able to recite or hear *Havdalah* until much later.[210]

The beverage

8a.   One may recite *Havdalah* with a beverage other than wine, provided that it is an important enough drink that in one's locality it is not drunk merely to quench thirst, but serves a social function and could grace the dinner table and be served to guests (See next paragraph for examples).[211]

8b.   Although it is ideal to recite *Havdalah* on wine, this is not always available in a hospital or safe for a patient to consume.   Some other alcoholic beverages acceptable for *Havdalah* include beer, brandy or another strong drink.[212] One may recite *Havdalah* on juice, ideally grape juice, but may also do so on orange or grapefruit juice, as well as cider.[213] Sweetened tea, coffee, or milk should only be used if one has nothing else available.[214] Neither water nor soft drinks should be used for *Havdalah*.[215]

The flame

9a.   Included in the *Havdalah* ceremony is the blessing made over a flame, "*Borei Meorei Ha-esh.*" Since one is not permitted to kindle an actual flame in the hospital, many authorities rule that one may use light from a clear electric incandescent bulb for this blessing.[216] However, one may not use an opaque or frosted light bulb (because the blessing should not be recited over a "flame" that is covered and not visible, even if one can see the light which radiates from it),[217] nor a fluorescent, LED or neon light (because they are not considered fire).[218]

9b.   If someone is blind, it is preferable for them to hear *Havdalah* recited by someone else. If no one else is available, the blessing "*Borei Meorei Ha-esh*" should not be recited.[219]

Fragrant spices

10a. While people often set aside a special container to make the blessing over fragrant spices, one may use any spice commonly found in the kitchen.[220] One should not use liquid perfume instead of spices.[221]

10b. If one is unable to obtain fragrant spices for the "*B'samim*" blessing, they may omit it and still recite the rest of *Havdalah*.   However, if they obtain spices later during the course of that Saturday night, they should make the blessing over smelling them.[222]

---

[209] Ibid., 299:1.
[210] *Mishnah Berurah* 296:21.
[211] *Shemirat Shabbat Kehilchatah* 60:3.
[212] Ibid., 60:4.
[213] Ibid., 60:5; *Lev Avraham* 14:37.
[214] Ibid., 60:6; *Lev Avraham* 14:37.
[215] Ibid., 60:7.
[216] Ibid., 61:32.
[217] Ibid., 61:31.
[218] Ibid., 61:32; *Nishmat Avraham OH* 296:1 (2).
[219] *Shulchan Aruch OH* 298:13; *Lev Avraham* 14:48.
[220] *Mishnah Berurah*, 297:10.
[221] *Shemirat Shabbat Kehilchatah* 61:12.
[222] Ibid., 61:3.

10c. If one is unable to smell, such as due to a cold, they should not recite this blessing. However, if one is with another person, they may ask that person to smell the spices and say the blessing, and then respond "Amen" to their blessing.[223]

One who is unable

11. If one is simply unable to get a clear light bulb or fragrant spices in the hospital, one may fulfill their obligation to recite *Havdalah* without either or both of these blessings.[224]

12. Although not all agree that women are obligated to make *Havdalah*, if there is no one available to make *Havdalah* for her, a woman may make *Havdalah* herself and drink the wine (or other suitable beverage).[225] A woman may also make *Havdalah* for a man if he is unable and there is no one else available to do so for him.[226]

13a. If one was unable to make *Havdalah* Saturday night, they should do so as soon as possible, up until sunset Tuesday night, at which point it may no longer be recited.[227]

13b. If one is making *Havdalah* after Saturday night, they should not recite the blessings over the flame or fragrant spices.[228]

14. It is preferable to wait and hear *Havdalah* in person rather than to hear it over the telephone,[229] but when no other solution exists, then one may fulfill their obligation by hearing *Havdalah* over the telephone and responding, "Amen" to the blessings.[230]

M. Food Preparation on Shabbat

One of the prohibited activities on Shabbat is cooking. This prohibition relates to both cooking raw food until it becomes edible and the act of warming foods, and particularly liquids, in many circumstances. At the same time, there is an obligation to enjoy Shabbat and eat enjoyable food on it (in accordance with the doctor's dietary instructions).

1. The *Shemirat Shabbat Kehilchatah* writes, "One may cook on Shabbat for a dangerously ill person who needs hot food to strengthen and refresh them if there is no suitable hot food available or the hot food which is available is not fresh enough for the patient. Similarly, if there is no hot water available, one may boil hot water on Shabbat for a dangerously ill patient who needs a hot drink."[231]

---

[223] Ibid., 61:5.
[224] *Shulchan Aruch OH* 297:1 & 298:1.
[225] *Shulchan Aruch OH* 296:8 & *Mishnah Berurah* 35; *Shemirat Shabbat Kehilchatah* 58:16. However, since a woman is not obligated to make the blessing on the light, it may be considered an unwarranted interruption, and she should thus either skip this blessing or say it after she has drunk from the *Havdalah* cup (*Shemirat Shabbat Kehilchatah* 61:24).
[226] *B'shvieli Beit Harefuah*, 23:1. In such a case Rav Shlomo Zalman Auerbach suggested that a man should first recite "Baruch Hamavdil Bein Kodesh L'chol" (*Shulchan Shlomo, Erchei Refua* vol. 1, 164).
[227] *Shulchan Aruch OH* 299:6.
[228] Ibid.
[229] *Guide for the Jewish Hospital Patient*, 22 (in the name of Rav Shlomo Zalman Auerbach).
[230] *Igrot Moshe OH* 4:91 (4).
[231] *Shemirat Shabbat Kehilchatah* 32:72. The *Shemirat Shabbat Kehilchatah* Hebrew edition 32 fn. 195 notes that if the food is not needed to strengthen and refresh the dangerously ill patient, only rabbinic prohibitions may be transgressed in the preparation of the food, not Torah prohibitions.

2.   One may not cook, or take part in any of the cooking process, for a patient who is not dangerously ill. However, one may ask someone who is not Jewish to cook or heat food or liquid for such a patient [see **pg. 24**, for an explanation of this concept].[232]

3a. A visitor, or any person who is not dangerously ill, may not eat any of the food cooked for a patient.[233] The only exception to this is if one needs to taste food for a dangerously ill patient to ensure that it is good for them.[234]

3b. If the food was not <u>cooked</u> on Shabbat, but was only <u>heated up</u> by someone who is not Jewish, the visitor may eat it on Shabbat once it has cooled down.[235] If the visitor has no other way of obtaining warm food on Shabbat, they may eat the remainder of pre-cooked food that was heated up on Shabbat by someone who is not Jewish for the sake of a patient, even while it is still hot.[236] On a *Yom Tov* (festival), however, food may be heated even for a visitor.

Opening Bags, Cans and Cartons

4a. Although it is ideal to open all cartons, cans, packaging etc. before Shabbat begins in order to avoid creating a new container on Shabbat, the *Shemirat Shabbat Kehilchatah* rules that, "One may tear open seals of the following kinds, (if one is very careful about the conditions contained in the next paragraph): paper seal covering the top of a bottle, paper wrapping around chocolate, the internal seal under the lid of a box or a jar of instant coffee (whether made of paper or other material); and the plastic or metal-foil top of a yogurt or sour-milk container.

The following conditions must be observed:

   a)   The seal or wrapping should be torn open in such a way that it is spoiled, and it goes without saying that one must not intentionally tear it in a manner which leaves even part of it fit for any use (as where one tears carefully along the edge of prize tokens printed on a wrapping). This condition is equally applicable whether one is tearing the wrapping or seal itself, or separated two pieces of paper or cardboard which are stuck together.
   b)   One must not tear through lettering or pictures."[237]

4b. Similarly, "Packets which are usually emptied of their contents and thrown away immediately upon being opened, such as packets of sugar, may be opened on Shabbat, even along a line specifically marked for that purpose, if indeed they are thrown away once opened. One should be careful not to cut or tear through lettering or pictures."[238]

---

[232] *Lev Avraham* 13:82 based on *Rema, Shulchan Aruch OH* 328:17.

[233] *Shemirat Shabbat Kehilchatah* 32:78; *Shulchan Aruch OH* 318:2

[234] *Shulchan Aruch OH* 318:2, *Mishnah Berurah* 11. This food, however, may be eaten by anyone immediately after Shabbat is over unless the food was cooked (not just warmed up) on Shabbat by someone who is not Jewish for a patient who is not dangerously ill, in which case there is a difference of opinion regarding the permissibility of someone else eating it after Shabbat (See *Nishmat Avraham OH* 326:62, pg. 461 for detailed discussion).

[235] Rabbi Zvi Goldberg, *"The Visitor's Halachic Guide to Hospitals"* Star –K Kashrus Kurrents, Vol. 29 no. 1 (Spring 2009), 2. This is because the prohibition is getting benefit from any forbidden labor on Shabbat, and once the food cools down there is no benefit from its being heated up.

[236] *Teshuvot V'Hanhagot* 3:363.

[237] *Shemirat Shabbat Kehilchatah* 9:11-12.

[238] Ibid., 9:4.

4c. Regarding opening a container for items such as tissues, cookies or cereal on Shabbat, the *Shemirat Shabbat Kehilchatah* writes, "Cartons of cut, folded toilet paper should not be opened by cutting along the special marking or tearing along a perforation, as is usually done in order to make a convenient slot to facilitate the removal of the paper, sheet by sheet. The carton should be ripped open and all of the paper removed."[239]

4d. The *Shemirat Shabbat Kehilchatah* also writes that, "Some authorities permit the opening of cans, bags, and paper packets which are not normally re-used, even without spoiling them, as long as: 1. One does not in fact intend to re-use them after removing their contents AND 2. One does not specifically intend to make a particularly neat opening for more convenient use."[240]

N. Treatment on Shabbat

1. One may carry throughout a hospital building even without preparing an "*Eruv Chatzeirot*."[241]

2a. A patient who is dangerously ill [see **pg. 16**, for an explanation of this concept] who is connected to an electric monitoring device, which keeps track of their blood pressure, heart rate, etc., may move in their bed on Shabbat as they please, even if this causes the numbers on the monitor to change.[242]

2b. A patient who is dangerously ill may even remove themselves from the monitor on Shabbat (if there is no one who is not Jewish available to do it for them) if they would like to get out of their bed for any reason (with the doctor's and nurse's permission). When the patient returns to their bed, they may reconnect themselves to the monitor (if a non-Jew is unavailable to do it [see **pg. 24**, for an explanation of this concept]) but should ideally do so in a manner different from what they would do during the week.[243]

3a. When one has an option of when to schedule a surgery, procedure, or childbirth it should ideally be done in the beginning of the week so that there is as little chance as possible of having to violate Shabbat for the patient's post-operative treatment.[244]

3b. However, one may choose to have a surgery at the end of the week in order to be treated by their preferred surgeon, to reduce the amount of time they have to spend waiting in the hospital (where they can more likely become ill), or if they are in pain and would like to have the surgery as soon as possible to relieve their suffering.[245] Similarly, if waiting to schedule a delivery of a baby will result in any danger to the mother or the fetus, it should be done as soon as the doctors recommend.[246]

---

[239] Ibid., 9:8.
[240] Ibid., 9:9.
[241] *Lev Avraham* 13;122; *Nishmat Avraham OH* 370:1.
[242] *Lev Avraham* 13:123.
[243] Ibid.
[244] *Shemirat Shabbat Kehilchatah* 32:35; 36:4.
[245] *Lev Avraham* 13:137.
[246] *Shemirat Shabbat Kehilchatah* 36:4.

3c. One should not have any surgery on Shabbat unless the doctor states that there is a pressing need and a delay could endanger the patient, in which case the surgery may take place on Shabbat.[247]

3d. If one must choose between having a procedure on Shabbat or *Yom Tov* (festival), it should be done on the *Yom Tov*. If it must take place on *Yom Tov*, one should choose the second day of the *Yom Tov* over the first.[248]

3e. The above notwithstanding, if a person has no choice and must undergo an operation at the end of the week, one may still violate Shabbat to do whatever is necessary for the patient, now that they are in the category of a patient whose life is in danger [see **pg. 16**, for an explanation of this concept].[249]

4a. One may allow any medical professional, Jewish or not, to perform necessary procedures for a dangerously ill patient on Shabbat, even if these acts would normally be considered violations of Shabbat. A dangerously ill patient who needs a procedure that could be safely delayed until after Shabbat may allow someone who is not Jewish to perform various necessary acts, such as an operation, take x-ray photographs, have a plaster cast filled, etc., on Shabbat.[250] As long as one is passive and not doing anything significant in the process, then he or she may allow someone who is not Jewish to take an x-ray or fill a cast even if they are not dangerously ill.[251]

4b. One whose condition is not life-threatening, however, should avoid treatment on Shabbat that can just as effectively be done on a different day of the week, such as certain preliminary x-rays, blood tests, or elective surgeries, as long as one's physician feels that it is safe to delay it. If there is a procedure that is necessary for the patient's health and welfare, one should allow a care-provider who is not Jewish to do it (unless a person is dangerously ill, in which case anyone, Jew or non-Jew, may carry out the procedure for the patient, as discussed in the previous paragraph).[252]

4c. One should not violate any Torah prohibitions on Shabbat in order to prepare for a surgery that will take place after Shabbat, unless delaying those preparations will significantly postpone an urgent procedure for this or another dangerously ill patient (though rabbinic prohibitions may be transgressed for this purpose, even for a non-dangerously ill patient, if it is not feasible to have the surgery at a different time).[253]

---

[247] *Lev Avraham* 13:213.
[248] Ibid. See also *Nishmat Avraham OH* 328:2 (9:2).
[249] Ibid.
[250] *Shemirat Shabbat Kehilchatah* 38:3. A Jew may not perform a procedure that constitutes a Torah prohibition if it is not essential on Shabbat, but if the procedure involves only a rabbinic prohibition, it may be performed, if necessary—though ideally in a way that differs from the normal manner if possible.
[251] Rabbi Gershon Bess, based on *Mishnah Berurah* 328:11. One does not have to remain entirely passive, but may adjust their body to enable the caregiver to help them, or put out their arm so that blood may be drawn, if necessary (*Nishmat Avraham OH* 328:3 (15)).
[252] *Guide for the Jewish Hospital Patient*, 22-23.
[253] *Nishmat Avraham OH* 328:49 (104:4).

5.   Although strenuous exercise is forbidden on Shabbat, one who needs to may engage in physical therapy (including the use of weights or springs) on Shabbat.[254]

6.   Hand sanitizers, such as Purell, are similar to liquid soap and may thus be used on Shabbat and festivals, even if they contain fragrances.[255]

Medicine

7.   There is a rabbinic prohibition against taking medicine on Shabbat.[256] This prohibition includes oral medication,[257] such as pills or liquids, and topical medication, such as medicinal lotions, ointments, sprays, suppositories, injections, or drops.[258] The regulations governing this prohibition are very intricate, but a brief overview of the subject is as follows:

8.   One who is dangerously ill [see pg. 16, for an explanation of this concept] may take medication on Shabbat for <u>any</u> ailment that they are suffering from.[259]

9.   One who is in the category of having a non-life-threatening serious illness [see **pg. 16**, for an explanation of this concept] may take all <u>necessary</u> oral medications on Shabbat.[260]

10.   Further exceptions to this prohibition may be made in the following cases:

•   If one is suffering from a painful ailment, the medicine may be mixed into food or drink before Shabbat.[261]

•   Medicine that must be taken daily, including Shabbat (and was already initiated before Shabbat), and will cause damage to the patient, or a relapse of the illness, if they do not take the medication on Shabbat.[262]

•   To preserve human dignity, e.g., to relieve a nasal discharge that is disturbing to other people.[263]

•   Non-oral medications or therapies may be administered if done in a manner differing from the way they would be done normally [see **pg. 23**, for an explanation of this concept].[264]

---

[254] *Nishmat Avraham OH* 328:42 (93). This is because most patients in need of physical therapy, such as massage used to free painful spastic muscles, or patients who have complete or partial paralysis of a limb and thus need certain exercises, are considered to be in the category of "danger to limb" or "incapacitating illness," for whom the prohibition against medicine on Shabbat does not apply. The same would apply to those patients who have recovered but are in need of daily physical therapy or else their condition would deteriorate back to one who has "danger to limb" or "incapacitating illness."

[255] Rabbi Dovid Cohen (in the name of Rav Gedalia Dov Schwartz), *Sappirim*, Issue 12 (Published by the CRC - Chicago Rabbinical Council, April 2008) 8, based on *Shemirat Shabbat Kehilchatah* 14:18. Bar soap, on the other hand, should not be used on Shabbat.

[256] *Shulchan Aruch OH* 328:1.

[257] Ibid., 328:37.

[258] Ibid., 328:20-25, 29-30.

[259] *Shemirat Shabbat Kehilchatah* 32:52, 56.

[260] *Shulchan Aruch OH* 328:37 Rema; *Mishnah Berurah* 328:121; *Shemirat Shabbat Kehilchatah* 33:4.

[261] *Shulchan Shlomo, Shabbat* 328:36.

[262] *Shemirat Shabbat Kehilchatah* 34:17 & fn. 77; *Lev Avraham* 13:190.

[263] Ibid., 34 fn. 52.

[264] Rabbi Gershon Bess based on *Mishnah Berurah* 328:102 & 130.

Taking Temperature on Shabbat

11. Use of a thermometer on Shabbat to take one's temperature is permitted for one who is ill, even if it is only a minor ailment.[265] According to Jewish Law, it is ideal to use the old-fashioned, mercury-type thermometer on Shabbat.[266]

12. A digital electronic thermometer is much more problematic according to Jewish Law because it works by turning on and off electrical circuits and causes numbers to be written on an electronic LCD display. Electric thermometers should thus preferably be used only for dangerously ill patient [see **pg. 16**, for an explanation of this concept], even if the caregiver who is operating it is not Jewish.[267]

13. Plastic strip and disposable chemical dot thermometers register temperature by changing colors depending on the design of each brand. If one can already make out the numbers or letters before the thermometer is used, it is permitted even to a patient with only a minor ailment, even if the color changes, since the letters were already there and using it added nothing, and it is only temporary writing. However, if the numbers or letters are not visible before it is used, it is forbidden because it is considered writing.[268] Nevertheless, if one is in a hospital and their temperature must be taken and this is the only type of thermometer available, it may be used.[269]

14. These guidelines and restrictions do not apply to one with a life-threatening illness or to a young infant for whom a fever can be life-threatening.[270]

Mental Anguish

15. The *Shemirat Shabbat Kehilchatah* writes, "It may happen that a dangerously ill person [see **pg. 16**, for an explanation of this concept] requests something which is unconnected with their medical treatment, but which would set their mind at rest or soothe them.

   a) One may not violate Shabbat by the infringement of a Torah prohibition in order to comply with such a request (except in the circumstances outlined in the next paragraph), but:

   b) One may infringe a rabbinical prohibition,[271] although here too, when possible, one should not perform the activity in the normal manner, but in a different way from that which one would adopt on an ordinary day of the week."[272]

16. "There are dangerously ill patients whose prospects of overcoming their illness and recovering their health depend on their mental state. In such cases, one should

---

[265] *Igrot Moshe OH* 1:128. Even though weighing and measuring is usually forbidden on Shabbat, the reason is that it is considered a weekday, professional/business type of activity, which taking the temperature of a patient is not (*Nishmat Avraham OH* 306:7(11)).
[266] *Chasdei Avraham*, vol. 2, 14:31.
[267] Ibid., 14:34. See, however, page 24 for further discussion.
[268] *Shulchan Shlomo, Erchei Refuah*, vol. 2, 143 & *Hilchot Shabbat* vol. 3, 311.
[269] *Shulchan Shlomo, Hilchot Shabbat* vol. 3, 312 (based on *Mishnah Berurah* 328:102).
[270] Rabbi Yisroel Pinchas Bodner, *Halachos of Refuah on Shabbos*, 353.
[271] See page 22 for some examples of rabbinic and Torah prohibitions.
[272] *Shemirat Shabbat Kehilchatah* 32:25.

be lenient and perform even acts prohibited by the Torah, if their omission might possibly result in a disturbance of the patient's mental equilibrium. One should also beware that the patient does not fall into a state of depression out of fear that they are not being properly taken care of."[273]

17. "One may violate Shabbat in cases of this kind, even when one has not been requested to do so by the patient."[274]

O. Pregnancy & Childbirth on Shabbat

Labor & Delivery

1. A woman during childbirth is considered to be in the category of a life-threatening seriously ill patient [see **pg. 16**, for an explanation of this concept], and the laws of Shabbat can be set aside for her (or the fetus) when necessary. However, unlike other patients in this category, since childbirth is a natural, physiological phenomenon, whenever possible the Shabbat prohibitions may only be set aside in an indirect or unusual manner or by someone who is not Jewish [see **pg. 23-24**, for explanations of these concepts].[275] No such variation from the normal manner should be done if it would result in a detrimental delay in doing what is necessary.[276]

2a. One may begin to suspend the laws of Shabbat where necessary from the moment she feels that the time has come for her to give birth. This moment is considered to have arrived once she begins feeling regular labor pains, even if it is doubtful whether or not birth is immediately imminent.[277]

2b. However, activities which can be delayed should not be performed in violation of Shabbat until the moment when:

   a) She is dilated to an extent which indicates that birth is imminent, or
   b) The water breaks, or
   c) The bleeding which can precede birth begins, or
   d) The patient is no longer able to walk between contractions.[278]
   e) Any other medically mandated reason.

Therefore, before one of these situations has arisen, one may only violate Shabbat to do something essential which is connected to the birth (such as transporting the patient to the hospital), but nothing unrelated to the birth itself (such as boiling water for the patient, activating an air conditioner, turning on a light, etc.) which may be done once one of these conditions has begun.[279]

---

[273] Ibid., 32:26.
[274] Ibid.
[275] *Shulchan Aruch OH* 330:1 & *Mishnah Berurah* 5; *Kitzur Shulchan Aruch* 93:2; *Lev Avaraham* 13:264; *Nishmat Avraham OH* 330:1(2 & 7).
[276] *Shemirat Shabbat Kehilchatah* 36:4.
[277] Ibid., 36:8.
[278] Ibid., 36:9.
[279] Ibid.

2c.   These rules apply both to a woman who is giving birth and to one who has had a miscarriage or abortion.[280]

3.   If there is a "false alarm" and it turns out that a woman has arrived at a hospital to give birth too early and she is thus discharged or refused admission on Shabbat, the *Shemirat Shabbat Kehilchatah* writes that she is not allowed to return home in a vehicle driven by a Jew. She may return in a vehicle driven by a non-Jew if:

   1)   There is nowhere comfortable in the vicinity of the hospital for her to stay until after Shabbat, **and**
   2)   Her home is within the "city limits."[281]

4.   If one is asked to sign something, such as a waiver or consent form for a specific treatment on Shabbat, see **pg. 38**, for guidelines. It is advisable to find out when one pre-registers if there is a chance that they may be asked to sign anything during the course of the delivery, and to sign it ahead of time so that they won't have to do so on Shabbat.[282]

5.   Before delivery, a woman may take a hot shower or bath and adjust the water temperature if she believes that the hot water will help the delivery[283] (though if possible this should be done by someone who is not Jewish).

Post-Partum

6.   After a normal vaginal delivery, a woman may not take a hot shower on Shabbat unless directed to do so for medical reasons. However, on a *Yom Tov* (festival), she may take a hot shower if she chooses,[284] (though ideally she should have someone who is not Jewish turn on the hot water if possible).

7a.   Once a woman has given birth, she is regarded by Jewish Law as a seriously ill patient whose life is in danger [see **pg. 16**, for an explanation of this concept] for a week after the birth.

7b.   This week is divided into two categories. For the first seventy-two hours from the time of the birth, one may violate Shabbat to do anything for the sake of the mother's health or to make her feel better, that someone with even minimal knowledge of medical matters sees as being necessary. This is the case even if there is no doctor or midwife available, and even if the mother herself doesn't think that she needs what is being done for her.[285]

7c.   Nevertheless, the manner in which one performs the forbidden act should be varied from the way one would do it on an ordinary weekday as much as possible,

---

[280] Ibid., 36:5 (assuming the miscarriage took place after more than forty days since the commencement of her pregnancy).
[281] Ibid., 36:10. "City limits" refers to the "*Techum*" (prohibition against traveling on Shabbat more than approximately 6/10th of a mile beyond the outer limits of the city one is in).
[282] Ibid., 36:9.
[283] Nachman Schachter, *Guide to Halachos*, edited and approved by Rabbi Moshe Heinemann, (Feldheim publishers), 41.
[284] Ibid.
[285] *Shemirat Shabbat Kehilchatah* 36:13. See also *Nishmat Avraham OH* 330:4 (12).

or if there is someone who is not Jewish available, it would be better if they did it [see **pgs. 23-24**, for explanations of these concepts].[286]

8. For the next ninety-six hours (four days),[287] Jewish Law continues to regard the mother as a patient whose life is in danger, but in this latter period one should not violate Shabbat for anything which the mother herself asserts that she does not need, even if non-professional laypeople think that the act in question is required for the patient (as long as the doctor or midwife does not say that the violation is necessary for her).[288] However, if there is no contrary medical opinion, then one may even rely upon a non-expert opinion to violate Shabbat for a mother in this category who sincerely requests.[289]

9. From day eight through the thirtieth day after the birth, the mother is no longer considered to be in danger, though she is still regarded by Jewish Law as a person who is ill [see **pg. 16**, for an explanation of this concept]. During this time, someone who is Jewish may transgress only a rabbinic Shabbat prohibition for the sake of the mother and it must be done in a manner different from the way it would be done on a weekday, or one may ask someone who is not Jewish to do anything necessary for the mother's health.[290]

10. In all of these situations it is permitted to directly ask somebody who is not Jewish to perform an action on behalf of an ill person, even one that is prohibited by the Torah, without the need to hint [see **pg. 24**, for an explanation of this concept].[291]

11. A woman who has a caesarean delivery is considered dangerously ill for as long as the doctors tell her she should be treated with extra caution (not limited to the above standardized time periods), after which she moves into the category of a patient who is not dangerously ill.[292]

12. If any potentially dangerous complications arise in the mother's condition anytime after the birth, she should once again be treated as a patient whose life is in danger.[293]

P. Nursing Mother on Shabbat

Cream may be dabbed on but not rubbed in because this action falls under the prohibited Shabbat labor of smoothing "*Memachaik*," which is the act of scraping or rubbing smooth a solid surface by side-to-side motions against a surface. A derivative of this prohibition is called "*Memarayach*," which is also a form of smoothing applicable to pliant, moldable substances. The primary prohibition is

---

[286] Ibid.
[287] *Shomirat Shabbat Kehilchatah* 39:15. These time frames are counted from the exact time of the birth, such that one may transition from one category to another even within the same Shabbat.
[288] Ibid., 36:14.
[289] Ibid.
[290] Ibid., 36:15.
[291] *Shulchan Aruch OH* 328:17, *Mishnah Beruah* 47; *Mishnah Berurah,* 330:16; *Shemirat Shabbat Kehilchatah* 36:15.
[292] *Shemirat Shabbat Kehilchatah* 36:16.
[293] Ibid., 36:15.

not transgressed simply by applying pressure, but by means of creating a smooth surface on wax or a thick ointment.[294]

1. If one needs creams or oils to make it easier for the baby to nurse, free-flowing oil may be applied, but thick cream may only be dabbed on and not rubbed in.[295]

"*S'chitah*" or squeezing falls under one of the categories of forbidden Shabbat labor known as "*Dosh*" or threshing, because just as this principle prohibits extracting a grain from its husk or peas from a pod, squeezing is the process of extracting liquid entity from its solid casing. Under certain conditions, the act of squeezing also transgresses the forbidden Shabbat labor of "*Melabain*" (the act of cleansing absorbent materials), because saturated moisture often cleanses a fabric as it is forced out of it. Squeezing or exerting pressure on a wet cloth or sponge is thus generally forbidden on Shabbat.

2. If the mother needs to clean herself before the baby nurses, she should not use wet absorbent cotton wool or gauze on Shabbat, even if it is held with forceps.[296] Instead, she should either use nylon (non-absorbent) swabs or if these are not available, she may first pour the liquid, such as water, alcohol or iodine, onto the part of the body concerned, and only afterwards wipe it dry with absorbent cotton wool, gauze or tissue.[297]

3a. Breastfeeding a child is completely permitted on Shabbat and Jewish holidays. However, expressing (pumping) milk into a receptacle for later use is prohibited on these days.[298]

Expressing milk is prohibited on Shabbat because, as mentioned above, one of the prohibited Shabbat labors is threshing, "*Dosh*," or the removal of grain kernels from their chaff. A derivative of this labor is called "*Mefarek*," which refers to extracting a food or liquid from its attachment or covering.

3b. Exceptions to this prohibition are made when the purpose of expressing the milk is either to relieve the mother's pain, or if the baby is unable to feed and there is a concern that by not expressing milk for an entire Shabbat, the mother will no longer be able to breast feed the baby who is in need of milk.[299]

3c. In these exceptions, milk should not be expressed into a vessel, unless it is in a way that ensures it cannot be used.[300]

---

[294] Ribiat, *39 Melochos*, 921.

[295] *Guide to Halachos*, 42. However, a patient who is dangerously ill (such as one who has or may develop pressure sores if not given preventative treatment) may apply cream or even ointment, if necessary, if it is completely rubbed into the body until it is entirely absorbed, because the Torah prohibition is only violated if it remains on the surface of the skin and is spread evenly (*Shemirat Shabbat Kehilchatah* 33 fn. 64; *Tzitz Eliezer* 7:67 (2) & 8:15 (14); *Nishmat Avraham OH* 328:22 (66)).

[296] *Shemirat Shabbat Kehilchatah* 36:17.

[297] Ibid., 32:59.

[298] Ibid., 36:18.

[299] Ibid., 36:21.

[300] Ibid.,36:20; see also *Mishnah Berurah* 330:32; *Shulchan Aruch OH* 328:34, *Beur Halachah s.v. "v'tanik."*

3d. If a mother is expressing milk in order to encourage a baby to begin nursing, she must express the milk directly into the baby's mouth.[301]

3e. If the baby does not normally drink formula, and its primary diet is its mother's milk, then for the sake of the baby it would also be permitted to express milk on Shabbat into a receptacle.[302] However, milk should not be expressed on Shabbat if it is to be used after Shabbat.[303]

4. Nursing caps may be used by mothers whose supply of milk is inadequate for their infants.[304]

5. If one uses an electric pump,[305] it should either be connected to a timer ("Shabbat clock")[306] or turned on by someone who is not Jewish.[307] If neither of these options is possible, then one may turn on the machine on their own in an abnormal manner, such as with the back of their hand or the back of a finger.[308]

Q. Care for Infants & Children

1. Any Shabbat prohibition may be set aside for the sake of a newborn (even in the case of a baby who will not be able to live for very long).[309]

2a. A child up to the age of nine or ten (depending on the stage of their development) generally requires special treatment and may thus always be classified in the category of a non-life-threatening serious illness [see **pg. 16**, for an explanation of this concept]. This applies both to preparation of food and to tending to the child's other needs which affect his or her health.[310]

2b. Therefore, one may ask someone who is not Jewish [see **pg. 24**, for an explanation of this concept] to do whatever is necessary for the well-being of a small child, even if it involves setting aside Torah prohibitions for their sake (such as cooking or turning lights on and off).[311]

Examples include expressing the milk directly into the sink or a cloth, or a contaminant like dish soap is put in the receptacle before expressing to render the milk unfit for use. If none of these exceptions exist, then one may not express milk, even if it will go to waste.

[301] Ibid., 36:20.

[302] Ibid., 36:22. This is only true if the baby is unable to nurse directly from its mother or is in the hospital and the mother has to bring fresh milk every day.

[303] *Lev Avraham* 13:292-293. If more milk is needed than can be expressed after Shabbat, formula should be given to the baby in addition to the mother's milk, unless the baby's health depends upon receiving its mother's milk.

[304] *The 39 Melochos*, 357. Nursing caps are specially designed cap-like devices placed over the nipples to collect droplets of milk that leak between each nursing.

[305] The *Shemirat Shabbat Kehilchatah* suggests that an electric pump may even be preferable to a hand pump which causes a new Shabbat violation with each pump (*Shemirat Shabbat Kehilchatah* 36: fn. 63), though Rabbi Ribiat advises using a hand pump instead of an electric device (*The 39 Melochos*, 356). See also *Nishmat Avraham OH* 328:35 (80).

[306] *Shemirat Shabbat Kehilchatah* 36:22.

[307] Some also rule that if possible the pump should be placed on the mother's breast before the machine is activated (*Guide to Halachos*, 42).

[308] *Lev Avraham* 13:291 (The *Lev Avraham* also quotes R. Ovadia Yosef, who suggests that one may activate the machine with the help of another person, so that it becomes a case of two people doing one act, and is thus only rabbinically prohibited on Shabbat).

[309] *Lev Avraham* 13:294.

[310] *Shemirat Shabbat Kehilchatah* 37:2.

[311] Ibid., 38:24.

2c. A child may be given any necessary medication, such as nose, eye or ear drops, syrups or tablets. The tablets may even be crushed and mixed with a drink if necessary.[312]

2d. However, each case must be judged on its own. If it is possible to satisfy the child's needs with something one already has and without violating Shabbat, one would certainly not be permitted to transgress even a rabbinic prohibition or ask someone who is not Jewish to do the act for them.[313] On the other hand, if the child is in fact seriously ill, one should follow the rules above in pg. 16 regarding doing whatever is necessary for the sake of a dangerously ill patient.

3. One may use baby wipes on Shabbat provided that they do not have to tear or separate attached towelettes. Furthermore, one must only make use of the moisture that is already on the surface of the cloth, and thus be careful not to apply pressure to avoid squeezing the contents out.[314]

4. Despite the prohibition against tearing, one may use disposable diapers on Shabbat and pull open their adhesive tabs, because the tab-shield is only a protective covering and is merely temporarily bonded.[315] Similarly, one may unfold a new diaper even if its lining is stuck or fused at the ends, because this fusing effect occurs unintentionally during production and packaging.[316]

5a. Lotion or baby oil should not be put on an absorbent material such as cloth or a cotton ball (because squeezing the liquid out of the cotton would constitute a violation of Shabbat). Rather, one may apply it by hand or by pouring it directly onto the baby's skin and only then gently wiping it with a cloth or towel (see explanation of this concept above in the section "Nursing Mother on Shabbat").[317]

5b. A thin oil with a liquid consistency may be applied to a baby's body, but a thick cream (such as Balmex, Desitin, or zinc oil) should not be smoothed onto a baby on Shabbat. If one wishes to smooth something of a thick consistency onto a baby, it should first be thinned out by adding a large quantity of oil[318] or it should simply be dabbed on the desired area instead of being smeared (see explanation of this concept above in the section "Nursing Mother on Shabbat").[319] Alternatively, one may apply a cream onto an infant if the cream will be completely rubbed into the skin so that it no longer creates a "smoothed surface."[320]

---

[312] Ibid., 37:9.

[313] *Shemirat Shabbat Kehilchatah* 37:2.

[314] *Guide for the Jewish Hospital Patient*, 37; *The 39 Melochos*, Rabbi Ribiat, 352 (though Rabbi Ribiat advises using tissues and water instead of baby wipes when possible).

[315] *The 39 Melochos*, 844. Rabbi Ribiat notes that if one wants to be strict, they can simply open and close the tabs before Shabbat to cause the bonding of the tabs to be classified as temporary.

[316] Ibid., 845-846.

[317] *Shemirat Shabbat Kehilchatah* 37:7.

[318] Ibid., 37:6.

[319] *Guide for the Jewish Hospital Patient*, 31.

[320] Rabbi Gershon Bess based on *Magen Avraham OH* 316:24 (quoted in *Mishnah Berurah* 316:49). (See paragraph 1.)

III. Festivals

Jewish holidays, such as Passover, *Shavuot, Sukkot, Rosh Hashanah,* and *Yom Kippur,* have restrictions and observances similar to those for Shabbat. For example, using electrical appliances, going to work, handling money, and writing—are all forbidden on festivals as well. The major differences between the two are that on festivals, cooking, lighting a fire from a pre-existing flame, and carrying in the public domain are generally permitted.[321] Some of the specific issues relevant to a hospital patient will be discussed below.

1. Some have the custom to avoid giving blood or having blood tests on the day before a festival, particularly *Shavuot.* However, a patient with any sort of medical need may do so.[322]

2a. Although on festivals one is technically permitted to light candles even after nightfall, this is only true if the flame is transferred from an already existing flame.[323] Since only electric candles can be used in the hospital, these may not be turned on after nightfall.

2b. For the same reason, there is no way to light electric candles on the second night of the festival. The only option would be for a patient's family member to light on their behalf at home. A person in the hospital for the festival would thus be considered unable to light and therefore exempt.

3a. As on Shabbat, if one was unable to make *Kiddush* in the evening, they should recite the evening *Kiddush* the next day.[324]

3b. Similarly, one who was unable to make *Kiddush* in the evening should simply say the "*Shehecheyanu*" blessing as soon as they are able, even if it is not while they are making *Kiddush.* If the entire day passes and one was unable to say it, one may even recite the blessing during "*Chol Hamoed.*"[325]

4. Unlike Shabbat, one may turn on a hot water faucet on festivals in order to wash one's hands and face (or other limited parts of the body).[326]

5a. Activating or deactivating an electric device on a festival is a rabbinic prohibition according to many authorities. One may, therefore, explicitly ask (i.e., without hinting) someone who is not Jewish to activate, deactivate or adjust the setting of any electrical device if the need derives from the necessity to perform a *Mitzvah,* enjoy the festival, significant monetary loss, slight illness, or another great necessity.[327]

---

[321] *Shulchan Aruch, OH* 495:1.
[322] Ibid., 468:10 & *Mishnah Berurah* 38.
[323] *Mishnah Beruah* 502:4.
[324] Ibid., 291:5.
[325] Ibid., 273:1; *Lev Avraham* 15:12.
[326] *Shemirat Shabbat Kehilchatah* 2:7; *Lev Avraham* 15:4.
[327] *Guide to Halachos* 47-48; *Shulchan Aruch OH* 502:1, 307:5.

5b. Similarly, a Jew may increase the setting on an infinitely adjustable dial (rheostat) on a festival, provided that the device is already activated and one is merely increasing an already existing flow of energy. For example, one may adjust the setting on a thermostat to cause the heater or air conditioning to run longer if it (including the condenser motor) is already running.[328]

6. The first and second days (as well as seventh and eighth) are both observed equally on each festival.[329] However, there are times when an action prohibited by rabbinic ordinance (and not the Torah itself) on the first day of a festival is permitted on the second day.[330] For example:

- If one is discharged from the hospital on a festival, it is preferable to leave (i.e., take a taxi driven by someone who is not Jewish) on the second (or eighth) day of the festival, rather than the first (or seventh).

- One may take medication on the second day of a holiday, even if they are just slightly uncomfortable.[331]

7. One who was unable to recite or hear "*Havdalah*" the evening on which the festival ended, should do so as soon as possible, but may do so the entire next day up until sunset of the day following the festival, but not later.[332]

A. *Chol Hamoed*

The holidays of Passover and *Sukkot* consist of two days at the beginning and two days at the end with complete festival restrictions and observances. The intermediate days between the beginning and end are known as "*Chol Hamoed*" and have far fewer restrictions.

1. Although on *Chol Hamoed* activities requiring professional precision are prohibited, one may perform any action necessary to treat even a minor ailment,[333] unless the matter could just as well be scheduled for after *Chol Hamoed*.[334]

2. Those who do not shave on *Chol Hamoed*, do not do so even if they were unable to shave before the festival due to an illness.[335] However, a patient may shave if this is part of his treatment.[336]

---

[328] *Guide to Halachos*, 49. Making sure the condenser motor is running is of no concern in a hospital.

[329] *Shulchan Aruch OH* 496:1.

[330] Ibid., 496:2 & *Mishnah Berurah* 7; *Lev Avraham* 15:1. Since the second days of the festivals are rabbinic, all prohibitions on these days are thus rabbinic, and therefore such a prohibition may be overridden in order to relieve even a minor ailment (*Shulchan Aruch OH* 496:2 & *Mishnah Berurah* 6-8). This is not true, however, on *Rosh Hashanah*, on which both days are treated equally.

[331] *Mishnah Berurah* 496:5; *Yom Tov Sheni Kehilchato* 1:22.

[332] *Mishnah Berurah* 273:16.

[333] *Shulchan Aruch OH* 532:2.

[334] *Igrot Moshe OH* 3:78.

[335] *Shulchan Aruch OH* 531:2-3.

[336] *Mishnah Berurah* 531:21; *Shemirat Shabbat Kehilchatah* 66 fn. 124.

B. *Rosh Hashana*

Rosh Hashanah, the Jewish New Year, is also commonly referred to as the Day of Judgment, as it marks the creation of humanity and is a time of reflection. It is a two-day holiday, with Sabbath-like restrictions, and one of its central observances is the sounding of the *Shofar*, a ram's horn.

1. Although rabbinic (not Torah) prohibitions may often be overridden for medical necessity on the second day of holidays (as discussed above), on *Rosh Hashanah* there is no difference between the first and second day.[337]

2. Although it is customary to have a new fruit or article of clothing in front of oneself when making the "*Shehecheyanu*" blessing on the second night of *Rosh Hashanah*, one may still recite the blessing even if one is unable to obtain such items.[338]

3. A man who lights holiday candles should recite the "*Shehecheyanu*" blessing when making *Kiddush*, but a woman should recite the blessing when she lights candles, and she should not repeat it if she makes *Kiddush* for herself.[339]

4. If one is unable to eat the various symbolic foods used for "*Simanim*" ("significant omens"), they may still recite the "*Yehi Ratzon*" prayers said over these foods.[340]

Shofar

4a. One who is unable to go to synagogue to hear the *Shofar* must try to ensure that someone can come to them so that they can hear at least thirty *Shofar* blasts.[341]

4b. A man who blows *Shofar* on behalf of other men should say the blessings of "*Lishmoa Kol Shofar*" and "*Shehecheyanu*" even if he has already fulfilled the *Mitzvah* of *Shofar* himself.[342] If he is blowing *Shofar* on behalf of a woman: If she is *Sephardi*, the blessings should not be said;[343] if she is *Ashkenazi*, the blessings should be said by the woman.[344]

5a. One may hear the *Shofar* even if they have not yet said their morning prayers.[345]

5b. Although one should not eat before hearing the *Shofar*, one who is ill and would find it difficult to go without food until they will be able to hear the *Shofar*, may make *Kiddush* and eat before hearing *Shofar* (although they should say the

---

337 *Shulchan Aruch OH* 496:2 & *Mishnah Berurah* 5-6.
338 Ibid., 600:2.
339 *Lev Avraham* 17:16.
340 *Nishmat Avraham OH* 583 (1). This is true even if one does not have the symbolic food in front of them at the time.
341 *Lev Avraham* 17:10.
342 *Shulchan Aruch OH* 585:2 *Rema; Shulchan Aruch OH* 589:6 *Rema*.
343 Ibid., 589:6.
344 Ibid., *Rema*.
345 Ibid.

morning prayers, or at least the blessings over the Torah and the first paragraph of *Shema*, before making *Kiddush*).[346]

C. *Yom Kippur*

Yom Kippur—the Day of Atonement, beginning eight days after *Rosh Hashanah*—is the holiest day of the Jewish calendar. Jews refrain from all eating and drinking for this entire day (commencing before sundown and concluding after nightfall the following day). Other pleasures, such as bathing or applying non-medical ointments, are also restricted.

Prayer

1. One who is unable to recite all of the *Yom Kippur* prayers should try to say at least the short confession ("*Viduy Katzar*"), "*Chatati, Aviti, Pashati*" and then ask God to cleanse and forgive them, and conclude with their own praise of God.[347]

2. One who is in an unclean environment may nevertheless recite the "*Viduy*" (confession) of *Yom Kippur* if they have no other choice, but without mentioning God's name.[348]

Eating

3a. Just as it is permitted, and even obligatory, to violate the laws of Shabbat in order to save life, so too it is a *Mitzvah* for a person whose life may be in danger to eat and drink (or transgress any other prohibition of the day) on *Yom Kippur*. Even a person who is not currently in mortal danger, but may become dangerously ill [see **pg. 16**, for an explanation of this concept] if they do not eat or drink, must eat or drink on *Yom Kippur*.[349]

3b. One who decides to be "strict" and fast despite the directive of their doctor and rabbi not to do so, is not considered pious but like a shedder of blood, about whom we apply the verse, "your blood, of your souls, I will demand an account."[350]

4a. A doctor's orders, irrespective of his or her religion, must be followed when they say that a patient must eat, even if the patient thinks that they can go without food.[351] If a doctor is not available, anyone who has any knowledge of medicine is trusted when they say that the patient must eat or drink to save their lives.[352]

---

[346] Ibid., 17:13; *Shemirat Shabbat Kehilchatah* 40:45.

[347] *Lev Avraham* 18:39; *Mishnah Berurah* 607:12.

[348] *Lev Avraham* 18:40, Rav Shlomo Zalman Auerbach adds that in such a case one should also not have in mind to be fulfilling the *Mitzvah* of "*Viduy*."

[349] *Shemirat Shabbat Kehilchatah* 39:1.

[350] *Mishnah Berurah* 618:5.

[351] *Shulchan Aruch OH* 618:1.

[352] *Mishnah Berurah* 618:1.

4b. If one is instructed to eat or drink, and they have time to consult with a rabbi, they must do so, particularly to find out if they should eat normal amounts or in measurements (see next section for explanation of this concept). However, if the case is urgent and life-threatening, and the physician has ordered the patient to eat without any delay, the doctor's orders must be followed.[353]

4c. The patient's own opinion that he or she is in need of food overrides that of a physician who disagrees,[354] unless the physician is of the opinion that food would actually do the patient harm.[355]

5. One should stay in bed in order to be able to fast on *Yom Kippur* rather than consume food or drink (even if only by measurements) so that they will be able to attend synagogue.[356]

6. A patient who is fed via an NG tube or PEG may continue to be fed in this manner on *Yom Kippur* (though one should not initiate feeding of this sort just in order to avoid the ruling of the doctor or rabbi regarding eating or drinking on *Yom Kippur*).[357]

7. Even one who is permitted to eat on *Yom Kippur* as a result of their poor health should eat only enough to provide the necessary nutrition and not consume any treats that they do not need to sustain them.[358]

8. One who only needs to drink but can avoid eating, for example to prevent a kidney stone, may drink (even beverages besides water, such as milk with sugar or fruit juice), but may not eat. If they must drink normal amounts they may do so; otherwise they should drink only in measurements.[359]

9. A diabetic patient receiving insulin, either by continuous infusion pump or by multiple injections, should fast on *Yom Kippur* if their doctor agrees that this will not put them in danger, by adjusting doses of insulin (by measuring the blood glucose levels).[360]

10. In any situation in which a patient must eat on *Yom Kippur*, the rabbi's and the physician's opinion must be sought regarding whether it will be sufficient to feed the patient in measurements (discussed below) or if the patient needs to eat regular amounts. Furthermore, one must also determine if it is sufficient to provide only beverages, or if the patient must eat food as well. There may also be times when one is permitted to eat once on *Yom Kippur* because of a great need, but they may still not eat any more after that.[361]

---

[353] *Lev Avraham* 18:5.
[354] *Mishnah Berurah* 618:4.
[355] *Aruch Hashulchan* 618:5-6.
[356] *Lev Avraham* 18:7.
[357] Ibid., 18:8-9.
[358] Ibid., 18:20.
[359] Ibid., 18:13.
[360] Ibid., 18:13.
[361] *Lev Avraham* 18:14; *Shemirat Shabbat Kehilchatah* 39:6.

Blessings

11. One who must eat on *Yom Kippur* does not recite *Kiddush* or use two loaves of bread, even if it is also Shabbat.[362]

12. Patients who must eat on *Yom Kippur* are obligated to wash their hands if they eat bread in the same manner as they would were it not *Yom Kippur*.[363]

13. One who is going to eat an amount of bread equivalent to the volume of an egg (approximately 1.9-2.95 fl. ounces) within nine minutes should also make the blessing over washing their hands. However, if one will not be eating this amount of bread, they should wash their hands without making the blessing.[364]

14. One who must eat on *Yom Kippur* makes the appropriate blessing before eating food, but when eating in "measurements" (as discussed below) they need only make the blessing once, and not repeat it every time they swallow food, unless they assumed that they would not need to eat any more.[365]

15. One who eats an amount of food equivalent to the size of an olive (approximately 1.1-1.5 ounces) within nine minutes must make the blessing after eating that food. If one ate bread, "*Yaaleh V'Yaavoh*" is inserted into the "*Birkat Hamazon*," although if one forgot, they need not repeat the "*Birkat Hamazon*."[366]

Taking Medication on *Yom Kippur*

16. One who has a non-life-threatening serious illness [see **pg. 16**, for an explanation of this concept] or may become ill without medication, may swallow pills if their doctor requires them to, but only if they can do so without swallowing any water along with it. It may be worthwhile to practice swallowing medication without water before *Yom Kippur*. If one is unable to do this and must take the medications, one may use a minimal amount of water to assist them in swallowing, but the flavor of the water should be made bad tasting by adding something bitter.[367]

17. However, one who is dangerously ill [see **pg. 16**, for an explanation of this concept] or may become so if they don't take their medication, may use undiluted water to help them swallow their medication if they are unable to do so without water.[368]

18. One who is healthy at the moment, but without medication will become ill, even not dangerously so (such as experience migraines or vomiting), may swallow a pill without water to prevent this condition. However, it is better to take the medication via a suppository, if possible.[369]

---

[362] *Mishnah Berurah* 618:29; *Lev Avraham* 18:26.
[363] *Lev Avraham* 18:25, Rav Shlomo Zalman Auerbach explains that one would wash their entire hand despite the prohibition against washing on Yom Kippur because this is not washing for pleasure.
[364] *Shulchan Aruch OH* 158:2.
[365] *Shemirat Shabbat Kehilchatah* 39:23.
[366] *Lev Avraham* 18:27; *Shemirat Shabbat Kehilchatah* 39:33.
[367] Ibid., 18:11-12; Dr. Abraham quotes Rav Shlomo Zalman Auerbach as allowing drops of soap to be added to the water to render it poor tasting, so that it is also considered drinking in an unusual manner, which is permitted for a non-dangerously ill patient. Some advise putting bitter-tasting Echinacea in water to use as the bitter drink (one should consult with a health care professional to determine if it is advisable to consume Echinacea on a fast day); others advise using something that is not fit for food, like Maalox, to get the medication down.
[368] Ibid., in the name of *Igrot Moshe OH* 3:91.
[369] Ibid., 18:12.

i. Eating in "Measurements"

Food

1. Though we have pointed out that one whose life may be endangered by fasting on *Yom Kippur* is obligated to eat, not all patients who are obligated to eat on *Yom Kippur* have the same exemption. Some patients' illnesses warrant only minimal eating or drinking as described below. This method is referred to as eating in "measurements" and it refers to eating less than a prescribed amount within a given period of time:

2a. The prohibition against eating on *Yom Kippur* is unique since "eating" isn't prohibited, but rather the Torah obligates "*Inuy*" or self-affliction (Leviticus 23:29). Eating an amount of food equivalent to a large date[370] is necessary to be considered culpable, because the rabbis ruled that any less than this does not put a person at ease and they are still "afflicted."[371]

   This amount is approximately 30 mL (or cc),[372] which is equivalent to just under one liquid ounce. One should measure before *Yom Kippur* how much food can be squeezed into a one-ounce whisky shot glass and eat just a bit under that amount.[373]

2b. It must be pointed out that these measurements apply to unique circumstances when one has specific permission to eat on *Yom Kippur* and only reference avoiding the punishment of "*Karet*" (spiritual excision) for eating on *Yom Kippur*. If it is not a life-threatening situation, partaking of even any amount of food or drink on *Yom Kippur*, regardless of how small, is prohibited by the Torah.[374]

3. One who is permitted to eat this minimal amount should preferably wait nine minutes (or at least 6-7 minutes)[375] from the time they finish the previous consumption until they begin eating or drinking again.[376] However, if the doctor determines that it is necessary for the patient to consume the food in a shorter span of time, one may do so.[377]

4. It is important to point out that these measurements govern the amount of food one eats, not the quality. One who must eat in this manner on *Yom Kippur* is thus advised to get the most out of their minimal consumption and choose foods with a lot of calories and nutrition to help sustain them throughout the day.[378] One should also discuss with their doctor what the ideal food or drink would be for them to consume in these small amounts.[379]

---

[370] *Shulchan Aruch OH* 612:1.
[371] *Mishnah Berurah* 612:1.
[372] *Nishmat Avraham OH* 612:1.
[373] Rabbi Gershon Bess.
[374] *Shulchan Aruch OH* 612:5 & *Mishnah Berurah* 612:11.
[375] *Aruch Hashulchan OH* 618:14.
[376] *Lev Avraham* 18:17; *Shulchan Aruch OH* 612:7.
[377] *Shemirat Shabbat Kehilchatah* 39:19; *Lev Avraham* 18:17. If one is unable to wait nine minutes between each food intake, or even 6-7 minutes, they should try to wait two minutes at the very least, if possible (*Nishmat Avraham OH* 612:4(6)).
[378] *Lev Avraham* 18:18.
[379] Ibid., 18:21.

5.   Since eating in measurements is preferable to eating larger amounts, one whose health condition and rabbinic ruling allow them to eat in measurements should begin doing so in the morning, to prevent their condition from deteriorating, thus forcing them to eat a larger amount of food.[380]

Beverages

6a.   The amount of liquid consumed on *Yom Kippur* to be considered culpable is more than a cheek-full, because the rabbis ruled that any less than this does not put a person at ease and they are still "afflicted."[381] For an adult this is generally about 40 mL of water,[382] which is about 1.3 ounces. The amounts of all liquids consumed, if one drinks different types, are added up and measured together for this purpose.[383]

6b.   One can ascertain his or her personal "cheek-full" by filling their mouth completely with water, expelling the water into a measuring cup and dividing that amount in half. This number is the amount held by one cheek, and the amount permitted is slightly less than this amount.[384]

6c.   It is advisable, but not obligatory, that all measurements be made before *Yom Kippur*.[385]

7.   One who is permitted to drink in measurements may drink beverages other than water, such as milk with sugar or fruit juice.[386]

8.   One should wait the same amount of time between drinks as is required for eating (paragraph 3 above), but if this is still insufficient for the patient, they should at least wait for a few moments (15-30 seconds)[387] between these minimal drinks.[388]

9.   Amounts of food and beverage are not combined, so that one may eat the minimal amount and then immediately drink the minimal amount.[389] However, if food, such as bread, has been soaked in a liquid, the measurements are combined so that one may still not eat more than 30 mL of this combined product.[390]

10.   If an item is normally chewed, then it is considered food, and if it is normally swallowed like a drink (such as porridge or sour cream), it is considered a beverage for these purposes.[391]

---

[380] *Shemirat Shabbat Kehilchatah* 39 fn. 69 (1979 edition).
[381] *Shulchan Aruch OH* 612:9.
[382] *Lev Avraham* 18:21.
[383] *Mishnah Berurah* 612:23.
[384] Rabbi Dovid Heber, *Star-K Kashrus Guide to Halachic Food Measurements*, http://www.star-k.org/kashrus/kk-issues-measurements.htm.
[385] *Mishnah Berurah* 618:21.
[386] *Lev Avraham* 18:18 in the name of Rav Shlomo Zalman Auerbach.
[387] Rabbi Gershon Bess.
[388] *Shemirat Shabbat Kehilchatah* 39:22.
[389] *Shulchan Aruch OH* 612:2.
[390] *Mishnah Berurah* 612:4.
[391] *Nishmat Avraham OH* 612:4(6).

ii. Pregnancy and Childbirth on *Yom Kippur*

1a. A pregnant woman who is well, and her fetus is well, must fast on *Yom Kippur* during all stages of pregnancy.[392] She should rest and avoid any strenuous activity or even going to synagogue. If she feels abnormal weakness she should drink in measurements, and if she needs, eat in measurements as well.[393]

1b. If she begins feeling regular contractions before she is full term, she should drink as much as necessary in order to stop the contractions. If she is full term and gets contractions, she should consult her obstetrician regarding drinking so as not to be dehydrated when giving birth.[394]

1c. Since a woman who has become pregnant following in vitro fertilization is more likely to miscarry during the first weeks after becoming pregnant, during these early stages of pregnancy she should drink in measurements.[395]

2a. From the time a woman is in active labor until seventy-two hours after she gives birth, she may not fast at all.[396]

2b. During this period, even if she and her doctor think that she is able to fast, she should eat, but in measurements.[397]

3a. After seventy-two hours following childbirth, i.e., from day four through day seven, the following rules apply:

- If the woman wants to eat and the physician doesn't disagree, or if the physician considers it necessary and she doesn't think that she needs to, then in both of these cases she should eat normal amounts.

- If she wants to eat but the physician does not consider it necessary, or if she is not sure and the physician does not say that she needs to eat, then she should eat only in measurements.

- If she says that she does not need to eat and the physician agrees, she should fast.[398]

3b. These time categories are based on the number of hours since giving birth. Therefore a woman's category may change during *Yom Kippur* itself.[399]

4. After the seven days following childbirth, the woman is classified as one who has a non-life-threatening serious illness [see **pg. 16**, for an explanation of this concept] until day thirty. A woman in this category must fast[400] unless her condition deteriorates and she or her doctor feels that it may become life-threatening, in which case she must eat.[401]

---

[392] *Lev Avraham* 18:30; *Shulchan Aruch OH* 618:1.
[393] *Lev Avraham* 18:30.
[394] Ibid.; Rabbi Gershon Bess.
[395] Ibid.
[396] *Shulchan Aruch OH* 617:4 & *Mishnah Berurah* 9, 13; *Mishnah Berurah* 330:10-11.
[397] Ibid., 617:4 & *Mishnah Berurah* 10; *Shemirat Shabbat Kehilchatah* 39:12.
[398] *Lev Avraham* 18:34; *Shemirat Shabbat Kehilchatah* 39:13.
[399] *Shemirat Shabbat Kehilchatah* 39:15.
[400] *Shulchan Aruch OH* 617:4.
[401] *Mishnah Berurah* 617:12.

5. The above rules apply equally in the case of a woman who has a live birth, a stillbirth, an abortion, or miscarriage more than forty days after becoming pregnant.[402]

6. A nursing woman is obligated to fast on *Yom Kippur*.[403] If the baby drinks formula, she should feed the baby with formula rather than break her fast. However, she may drink (but not eat) in measurements if she would not otherwise have sufficient milk for her baby and the baby is entirely dependent on her milk for its sustenance, thus putting the baby's life in danger.[404] She should try to avoid this situation by drinking large quantities of liquid before *Yom Kippur* begins.[405]

D. *Sukkot*

Sukkot, the Festival of "Tabernacles," is a joyful holiday celebrated five days after Yom Kippur. It begins before sunset and extends until nightfall seven days later, when *Shemini Atzeret/Simchat Torah* begins. The first two and last two days of this period have Sabbath-like festival restrictions. During the first seven or eight days of this holiday, one eats and dwells in a Sukkah (temporary outdoor structure) and recites blessings over the Four Species (citron, palm branch, myrtle, and willow branches).

1a. One who is ill is not obligated to dwell in a *Sukkah*.[406] This is because one is supposed to dwell in a *Sukkah* the way they would dwell in their home. Since hospitalized patients are not dwelling in their homes, they are exempt.[407] This exemption not only applies to one whose life is in danger, but also to a person suffering from a mild ailment [see **pg. 16**, for an explanation of this concept], who need not eat in the *Sukkah*[408] if eating elsewhere is more comfortable.[409]

1b. One who is assisting a patient is also exempt from dwelling in a *Sukkah* during the time that the patient requires him or her.[410] If the patient's life is in danger and they need constant supervision, one who is attending to them would remain exempt at all times.[411]

2. One should not eat before fulfilling the *Mitzvah* of shaking the *Lulav*.[412] However, one who is ill and would find it difficult to go without food until they will be able to do this *Mitzvah*, may eat before they pray, but should at least recite the blessings of the Torah and the first paragraph of the *Shema* (and recite *Kiddush* if it is Shabbat or *Yom Tov*) before eating.[413]

---

[402] *Shemirat Shabbat Kehilchatah* 39:16.
[403] *Shulchan Aruch OH* 617:1.
[404] *Shemirat Shabbat Kehilchatah* 39:18.
[405] Ibid.
[406] *Shulchan Aruch OH* 640:3.
[407] *Mishnah Berurah* 640:6.
[408] *Shulchan Aruch OH* 640:3.
[409] *Mishnah Berurah* 640:9.
[410] *Shulchan Aruch OH* 640:3.
[411] *Mishnah Berurah* 640:11.
[412] Ibid., 692:15.
[413] *Lev Avraham* 19:13.

3a.   One who does not have any use of their hands should take hold of the *Lulav* and *Etrog* with their arm if possible.[414] If one has only one hand, they should take hold of the *Lulav* (along with the *Hadassim* and *Aravot*) with that hand and hold the *Etrog* with the arm opposite it. If one is unable to take hold of the *Etrog* with their arm, then they should take the *Lulav* and *Etrog* individually in succession, first the *Lulav* by itself and then the *Etrog* by itself, in their good hand (regardless if that is the right or left hand).[415]

3b.   One whose arm is paralyzed, but is able to take hold of the *Lulav* and *Etrog* with some assistance from another person, may fulfill the *Mitzvah* in this manner.[416]

4.   Although one should stand while making the blessings "*Al Netilat Lulav*" and "*Shehecheyanu*,"[417] if one is unable to stand, they may say it while sitting.[418]

5.   If possible, one should remove any Band-Aids or bandages from their hands before performing the *Mitzvah* of taking the *Lulav* and *Etrog*, but if they are unable to, or if it is inadvisable to do so, they may nevertheless perform the *Mitzvah* and say the blessings with them on.[419] Similarly, one whose hand is encased so that they can only hold the *Lulav* or *Etrog* with their fingers, may nevertheless perform the *Mitzvah* and say the blessings.[420]

E. *Chanukah*

Chanukah, the Jewish festival of rededication, also known as the "festival of lights," is an eight-day minor holiday in the winter, on which all types of "work" that are prohibited on Shabbat and most other holidays are permitted. *Chanukah* is generally observed by lighting candles in the evening and reciting additional prayers of thanksgiving.

Electric Lights

1.   According to most opinions, one does not fulfill the *Mitzvah* of lighting *Chanukah* candles with electric lights.[421] However, a hospitalized patient who has no alternative should perform the *Mitzvah* of lighting the *Menorah* with electric lights, but should not recite the blessings.[422]

---

[414] *Shulchan Aruch OH* 651:4.
[415] *Mishnah Berurah* 651:23.
[416] *Lev Avraham* 19:13.
[417] *Shulchan Aruch OH* 651:4 *Rema*.
[418] *Mishnah Berurah* 651:27.
[419] *Lev Avraham* 19:13.
[420] Ibid.
[421] Although this is the general practice, *Lev Avraham* 23:2 quotes a ruling of Rav Eliyashiv and Rav Shlomo Zalman Auerbach that if one is in a difficult situation and has no other choice, they may make a blessing on electric lights, such as flashlights, as long as they are battery powered and have enough energy left in the batteries to last the entire time that the candles must stay lit. A blessing should not be said on a *Menorah* that is plugged into an electrical outlet.
[422] *Lev Avraham* 23:1. The rules of lighting a *Chanukah Menorah* differ from those of lighting Shabbat candles because on Shabbat the goal is to bring illumination to the room in honor of Shabbat, whereas on *Chanukah* we

Location of Lights

2a. When lighting an electric *Menorah* in a hospital room, it is best to place it in a spot where one does not normally put lights so that it is clear that it is there for the sake of the *Mitzvah*.[423]

2b. It is best to light one's *Menorah* near the window in order to publicize the miracle. This is so even for one who normally lights their *Menorah* by their front door, since this is generally not feasible in a hospital.[424]

2c. There is a principle that the kindling is the performance of the *Mitzvah*, and not the placing of the light.[425] Therefore, a patient who is confined to their bed and cannot get up to kindle the *Chanukah* lights by the window should not light them next to their bed and have someone move them. Rather, another person should kindle them in the correct place on behalf of the patient or they should be kindled by the bedside and left there.[426]

Spouse on Behalf of Patient

3. The *Mishnah Berurah* writes, "When one's wife kindles *Chanukah* lights in his home he fulfills his obligation with her kindling, even if he is in a place that is far away from his home."[427] Therefore, the spouse of a hospitalized patient should light the *Chanukah* lights at home and bear in mind to include their husband or wife in the *Mitzvah*.[428]

F. *Purim*

Purim is a one-day annual minor holiday commemorating the miracle recounted in the Biblical book of Esther. On this holiday, traditionally observant Jews are allowed to do the types of "work" that are prohibited on Shabbat and most other holidays, but there are a number of special *Purim* obligations that many Jewish patients will want to fulfill.

---

1. A patient who is unable to attend synagogue to hear "*Parshat Zachor*" should read it from a Torah scroll without a blessing or, if this is not possible, read it from a printed *Chumash*.[429]

---

attempt to reenact the miracle of the *Menorah* that occurred with burning wicks and oil.
[423] Ibid.
[424] *Chasdei Avraham* vol. 3, 23:2.
[425] *Shulchan Aruch OH* 675:1.
[426] *Lev Avraham* 23:3.
[427] *Mishnah Berurah* 677:2.
[428] *Lev Avraham* 23:6.
[429] Ibid., 24:1.

2a. One who is healthy may not eat a meal before hearing the reading of the *Megillah* on *Purim* eve, even if the fast has been difficult.[430] However, a light snack may be eaten if necessary.[431]

2b. If waiting until someone comes to read the *Megillah* in one's room on *Purim* night will be too difficult, one may arrange to hear the *Megillah* during the afternoon before Purim if possible, as long as it is after "*Plag Haminchah*" (an hour and a quarter before sunset).[432] They may then break their fast upon *Halakhic* nightfall ("*Tzeit Hakochavim*").

2c. If one needs to eat before hearing the *Megillah*, and a light snack will not be sufficient, the patient may eat as needed but should ask to be reminded to hear the reading of the *Megillah* after their meal.[433]

Megillah

3. A patient who is unable to attend synagogue to hear the *Megillah* should try to hear it with a *Minyan*. [434]   If this is not possible they should have someone read the *Megillah* for them, or they should read it themselves, from a kosher *Megillah* scroll and recite all the blessings before the reading,[435] but not the blessing after.[436]

4a. One who has already fulfilled the *Mitzvah* of reading the *Megillah*, and reads it again for the sake of someone who was unable to attend synagogue, may recite the blessing over reading the *Megillah* again.[437]

4b. However, if the *Megillah* is being read for women only, the blessing should be changed to "*Lishmoa Megillah*" (to hear) instead of "*Al Mikra Megillah*" (over the reading of), because women are obligated only to hear the *Megillah* read, but not to read it themselves. It is ideal for one of the women in attendance to recite the blessings instead of the man who is reading if he has already fulfilled his obligation.[438]

5. One who is in the hospital and is unable to find anyone who can read the *Megillah* for them and is too weak to read it on their own, may hear the *Megillah* over the phone and respond "Amen" to the blessings, even though in normal circumstances this is not permitted.[439] If even this is not an option, one should read the *Megillah* from a printed text without reciting any blessings, though this would not fulfill the *Mitzvah* to hear the *Megillah*.[440]

---

430 *Shulchan Aruch OH* 692:4 *Rema*.
431 *Mishnah Berurah* 692:14.
432 Ibid., 692:14; *Beur Halachah* s.v. "*Miplag*."
433 Ibid., 692:16.
434 *Shulchan Aruch OH* 690:18.
435 *Mishnah Berurah* 692:8.
436 *Shulchan Aruch OH* 692:1 *Rema*; See also *Nishmat Avraham OH* 690:1.
437 *Shulchan Aruch OH* 692:3.
438 *Mishnah Berurah* 692:11; *Chasdei Avraham* Vol. 3, 24:4; See *Nishmat Avraham OH* 689:3 who notes that in some *Sephardic* communities the *Megillah* is read for women without a blessing while in others the *Megillah* is read for women with the same blessing of "*Al Mikra Megillah*," that is recited when the *Megillah* is read for men.
439 *Chasdei Avraham* vol. 3, 24:6; *Guide for the Jewish Hospital Patient*, 33. This should also apply to watching the live *Megillah* reading on the patient's television set.
440 *Shulchan Aruch OH* 691:10.

Mitzvot of *Mishlo'ach Manot* and *Matanot La-Evyonim*

6a. One who is a patient in the hospital is still obligated to fulfill the other *Mitzvot* of *Purim* if possible. The patient should arrange for them to be performed on their behalf by another person.[441]

6b. If possible, one would be allowed to trade a portion of their meal with another patient (assuming they both receive kosher meals and do not have any unique dietary restrictions)[442] to fulfill the *Mitzvah* of *Mishlo'ach Manot*.[443]

G. Passover

Passover is one of the most widely observed Jewish holidays. This eight-day springtime festival commemorates the exodus of the Jewish slaves from Egypt and their subsequent freedom. During Passover, no bread or other products of grain fermentation may be eaten or even owned by a traditionally observant Jew. Sabbath-like festival restrictions are observed on the first two and last two days of the holiday.

"*Chametz*" is any food product made from wheat, barley, rye, oats, spelt, or their derivatives, which has leavened (risen) and/or which has come into contact with water for more than 18 minutes.

"*Kitniyot*," sometimes referred to generically as "legumes," include rice, corn, soy beans, string beans, peas, lentils, mustard, sesame seeds and poppy seeds. Even though *kitniyot* cannot technically become *Chametz*, Ashkenazi Jews do not eat them on Passover.

Searching for & Selling *Chametz*

1. The owner of a space, or tenant if the premises are rented, is required to search for *Chametz* on the night of the fourteenth of *Nissan*.[444] One who is unable to be at home at this time may appoint a representative to do the search for them.[445]

2. If one does not have anybody available to do the search for them, and they will be leaving their home before the fourteenth (but within thirty days of Passover), then they must do the search and nullification of *Chametz* the night before they leave their house, without reciting the blessing.[446]

---

[441] *Lev Avraham* 24:6.
[442] See *Nishmat Avraham OH* 695:1 that one would not fulfill the *Mitzvah* of *Mishlo'ach Manot* by sending food that the recipient is not permitted to eat due to their illness.
[443] Ibid.
[444] *Shulchan Aruch OH* 437:1.
[445] *Shulchan Aruch OH* 432:2 & *Mishnah Berurah* 8, 11; *Shulchan Aruch OH* 436:1. This representative is ideally an adult male, but may also be a woman or a responsible child, *Mishnah Berurah* 436:1, 437:18-19.
[446] *Shulchan Aruch OH* 436:1.

3. One is not required to do a "*Bedikat Chametz*" (search for leavened products) in their hospital room since they do not own it, but they should check all of their possessions to make sure that they do not have any *Chametz* amongst their belongings, and one should also check any areas designated for the patients' personal use, such as closets, the night table, and drawers. A blessing would not be made on this search.[447]

4. A person can do "*Bittul Chametz*" (nullification of leavened products) in their hospital room, and make a statement to the effect that they do not intend to automatically acquire any *Chametz* that might be in their hospital room. If they find *Chametz* in the room over Passover, they can assume it is abandoned. If they would like to avoid inadvertent consumption, they can cover it on the holiday, or destroy it on *Chol Hamoed*.[448]

Seder

1a. One who is unable to have an entire *Seder* on Passover night or is busy taking care of a patient who is dangerously ill, should at least:

- Recite *Kiddush* and try to drink minimally 86 grams (3.03 ounces) of the cup while reclining.

- Then recite the "*Avadim Hayinu*" ("we were slaves") section of the *Haggadah*, since it encompasses the primary obligation of telling the story of the Exodus. If one has a little more time it is ideal to recite the "*Rabban Gamliel Haya Omer*" ("*Rabban Gamliel* used to say") section as well.

- Then drink a second cup while reclining after saying the blessing of "*Asher Ga'alnu*."

- Then wash their hands and make the blessing of "*Al Netillat Yadayim*."

- Then take three *Matzot* (two will suffice if they don't have three), say the blessings of "*Hamotzi*" and "*Al Achilat Matzah*" and eat about 17-20 grams (0.6-0.7 oz.) within about 4-5 minutes, while reclining.

- If more time is available, one should eat some *Maror* after reciting the appropriate blessing, without reclining.

- At this point one may eat their meal and then the second *Matzah* for *Afikoman*, followed by the grace after meals, the blessing for the third cup and the blessing said after drinking the cup.[449]

1b. If one would not have time to eat *Matzah* twice, before the meal and again for *Afikoman*, they should:

---

[447] Rav Yiztchak Zilberstein, *Torat Hayoledet* 277.
[448] *Shulchan Aruch OH* 446:1, *Mishnah Berurah* 435:5.
[449] *Lev Avraham* 20:1 (1).

- Eat their entire meal without *Matzah*.

- At the end of the meal wash their hands without saying the blessing of "*Al Netillat Yadayim.*"

- Say the blessings of "*Hamotzi*" and "*Al Achilat Matzah*" and then eat the *Matzah* while reclining for the sake of both the *Mitzvah* of *Matzah* and the *Mitzvah* of *Afikoman.*

- One should then say the grace after meals and if possible, drink another cup and make the blessing after that.[450]

1c.   If one has the strength to continue before midnight, they should drink the third cup (if they have not yet done so) with its appropriate blessing, say *Hallel* and then drink the fourth cup while reclining, and conclude with the blessing after drinking wine/grape juice. If possible, one should say the prayers of "*Nishmat*" and "*Yishtabach*," as well as whatever else they had to skip in the *Haggadah.*[451]

2.   One who may become busy taking care of a patient or for some reason does not think that they will be able to do the entire *Seder* at once, should make a condition from the outset that when they eat the *Matzah*, if they are interrupted and unable to return to their *Seder*, then the *Matzah* that they are eating now should also be counted as fulfilling the *Mitzvah* of *Afikomen*. But if they are able to return to the *Seder* before midnight, then the *Matzah* which they already ate should be considered a fulfillment of the *Mitzvah* of *Matzah*, and the *Matzah* they eat at the end of the meal (before midnight) will be to fulfill the *Mitzvah* of *Afikomen*. If they diverted their attention from the meal during the break, they will have to wash their hands and make "*Hamotzi*" again.

3a.   If one is needed to care for a dangerously ill patient, they must do so and forgo their performance of the *Seder*.[452] If one was unable to perform the *Seder* until after midnight, they may still do all of the *Mitzvot* of the night, but since it is questionable whether they are actually fulfilling the *Mitzvot* at this time, they do not say the blessings of "*Al Achilat Matzah*" or "*Al Achilat Maror*" on the *Maror*. In this case one should drink all four cups, but only say the blessings on the first and third cups.[453]

3b.   If one was unable to do any of this and the entire night passes without having performed the *Seder*, it cannot be made up or performed at another time.[454]

---

[450] Ibid., 20:1 (2).
[451] Ibid., 20:1 (3-4).
[452] Ibid., 20:1.
[453] Ibid., 20:1 (7).
[454] *Magen Avraham OH* 485:1; *Shaarei Teshuvah* 482 intro.

Wine, *Maror* & *Matzah*

4a. Although the "four cups" during the *Seder* are ideally fulfilled by drinking wine,[455] one may use grape juice[456] or another suitable beverage,[457] such as tea, coffee or juice if they are unable to drink wine or grape juice.[458]

4b. One who is responsible for tending to a patient should not drink wine so that their concentration is not impaired.[459]

5. One who is ill or very picky may choose any of the acceptable options for *Maror* that they prefer, such as romaine lettuce rather than horseradish, and may eat it little by little over the course of a few minutes. Even if they don't like *Maror*, they should try their best to eat it. However, if it would be damaging to their health, they should try to simply eat a tiny bit or at least chew some in their mouth to get a taste of the bitterness (though in this case they would not make the blessing).[460]

6. One who has difficulty chewing, swallowing, or digesting *Matzah* in its normal state, may crush it into small pieces and eat it this way at the Seder. If eating it dry is too difficult, one may soften the *Matzah* by dipping it into water, or when absolutely necessary, in another beverage (but one must make sure that the *Matzah* does not disintegrate and liquefy).[461]

7. If one vomits after eating *Matzah*, *Maror*, or drinking one of the cups, since they have already swallowed it they have fulfilled the *Mitzvah* and do not need to eat or drink again. However, if one has regurgitated all the *Matzah* that they ate, they will be unable to recite the grace after meals.[462]

8. If drinking the cups, or eating *Matzah* or *Maror* will cause a patient to have internal illness or the need to lie down, they are exempt from the *Mitzvah* and should not do so.[463]

9. One who is fed through a PEG or NG tube will be unable to fulfill these *Mitzvot*, but if possible they may listen to someone else make the appropriate blessings and have in mind to fulfill the *Mitzvot* in this manner.[464]

10. One who has celiac disease and cannot eat gluten or any wheat may not eat *Matzah* if they know it will lead to illness, but should instead eat oat *Matzah* if possible. However, if this person does occasionally eat bread during the year, they should then have a *Seder* without *Matzah*, but at the end wash their hands

---

[455] *Shulchan Aruch OH* 472:10.
[456] *Lev Avraham* 20:1 (1) fn. 2 & 20:5.
[457] *Mishnah Berurah* 472:37.
[458] *Guide for the Jewish Hospital Patient* 35.
[459] *Lev Avraham* 20:1 (1) fn. 2.
[460] Ibid., 20:2 based on *Mishnah Berurah* 473:43.
[461] Ibid., 20:3 based on responsa *Binyan Tzion* 29 and *Mishnah Berurah* 461:18.
[462] Ibid., 20:4.
[463] Ibid., 20:6; *Mishnah Berurah* 472:35; *Shemirat Shabbat Kehilchatah* 32 fn. 73; It should be pointed out that if one is not sick and one only dislikes or is mildly harmed by these substances, he or she must nevertheless consume them (*Shulchan Aruch OH* 472:10).
[464] *Lev Avraham* 20:7.

without reciting a blessing, then say the blessings of "*Hamotzi*" and "*Al Achilat Matzah*" and then eat the minimum amount of *Matzah* (as described in paragraph 1a above) while reclining, for the sake of both the *Mitzvah* of *Matzah* and the *Mitzvah* of *Afikoman*.[465]

11.   If one is unable to recline, they are not obligated to do so.[466]

12.   One who is unable to eat the proper amount of *Matzah* or *Maror* within the minimum time (discussed above) should eat it without reciting the appropriate blessing.[467] If their doctor advises them not to consume *Matzah*, *Maror* or wine and they do so anyway, they have committed a transgression and not a *Mitzvah*.[468]

Chametz & Kitniyot

13.   A patient who is not seriously ill may not take, or even have in their possession, any pleasant-tasting medicine such as lozenges or syrup, if they contain any *Chametz* at all.[469]

14.   However, a non-seriously ill patient may swallow pills or capsules that are unpalatable, and may have them in their possession, even if they contain a *Chametz* ingredient.[470] (There are many Israeli-produced medicines that are certified Kosher for Passover.)

15a.   A patient who is dangerously ill, or even just potentially so [see **pg. 16**, for an explanation of this concept], may eat or drink *Chametz* food if they are specifically required by the physician for one's healing, even if it is not certain that it will cure the patient, unless there is a non-*Chametz* alternative. One is obligated to consume *Chametz* if this is what their doctor has prescribed for the sake of saving their life.[471]

15b.   Since medications containing *Chametz* may sometimes be taken on Passover when necessary, one should consult their physician and rabbi to discuss their case. For example, all medications for a heart condition, diabetes, abnormal blood pressure, stroke, kidney disease, lung disease, depression, epilepsy, the immune system (transplant anti-rejection), and cancer treatment (including precautionary) may be taken on Passover. Furthermore, all prescription medication taken on a regular basis for chronic conditions should only be changed with the consultation of one's physician (if one cannot reach his or her physician, they should continue to take their regular prescription and not change). Some examples of such chronic conditions include any psychiatric condition, prostate condition, Crohn's disease, colitis, high cholesterol, Parkinson's disease, anemia, multiple sclerosis, thyroid condition, and asthma.[472]

---

[465] Ibid., 20:9.
[466] Ibid., 20:10.
[467] *Guide for the Jewish Hospital Patient* 35.
[468] *Nishmat Avraham OH* pg. 342 (8); *Maharam Shik OH* 260; *Minchat Yitzchak* 4:102 (2).
[469] *Lev Avraham* 20:12.
[470] Ibid.
[471] Ibid., 20:11.
[472] Rabbi Gershon Bess, *A Passover Guide to Cosmetics and Medications*, Kollel-Los Angeles 2011, Intro.

16. Although *Ashkenazim* do not eat *Kitniyot* (rice, beans or any leguminous vegetables) on Passover, a non-seriously ill patient or a child suffering from a condition, such as diarrhea, whose doctor says they must eat one of these products, like rice or corn flour, may do so.[473]

17. Since most pills and capsules are made of starch or amylum which are made of *Kitniyot*, but do not contain any *Chametz* (and even if they do contain *Chametz*, it is probably unpalatable), even a non-seriously ill patient may take them on Passover.[474] One should not be strict and discontinue necessary medication on Passover if they have been advised by a doctor to take it on Passover, particularly if there is any chance that discontinuing the medication may lead to any possible danger to the patient.[475]

18. Alcohol based hand sanitizers, such as Purell, typically contain ethyl alcohol, which may be *Chametz*. However, since it is inedible (like liquid soap) and the alcohol content is denatured, these products may be used on Passover.[476]

19. A patient, even if not dangerously ill, whose custom is not to eat *Gebrukts* (Matzah that has absorbed liquid) on Passover, may nevertheless eat it if they have nothing else available.[477]

Medicine on Passover (Summary)[478]

A. A patient who is (or may become) **seriously ill**:

- May eat or drink products containing *Chametz* if this is necessary to cure the patient, even if they will not certainly cure him or her, if one cannot easily obtain a *Chametz*-free alternative.

- Not only is this permissible, but it is obligatory since it can be categorized as life-saving.

B. A patient incapacitated but **not dangerously or seriously ill**:

We must distinguish between eating *Chametz* in the normal manner when the product has a good flavor (palatable) and those medications which are not eaten in the normal manner and provide no flavor. We also distinguish between products in which the *Chametz* itself gives a good flavor to the item, and those in which the flavor comes from non-Chametz sugar mixtures and the *Chametz* itself does not taste good and is not edible by itself. Because there are numerous opinions and relevant factors, one should consult their rabbi for specific questions related to taking medicine on Passover. A general summary of the conclusions of the leading authorities in Jewish law is as follows:

---

[473] Ibid., 20:13 based on *Mishnah Berurah* 453:7.
[474] Ibid., 20:14.
[475] Ibid., based on *Mishnah Torah, Yesodei Hatorah* 5:8, *Shulchan Aruch YD* 155:3 & *Shach* 13, *Chazon Ish OH* 116:8, *Minchat Shlomo* 1:17, *Shemirat Shabbat Kehilchatah* 40 fn. 169.
[476] Rabbi Dovid Cohen, *Sappirim* (Published by the CRC - Chicago Rabbinical Council), April 2008, Issue 12 pg. 4 in the name of Rav Gedalia Dov Schwartz.
[477] Personal communication with Dr. Abraham S. Abraham.
[478] All based on *Nishmat Avraham OH* 466:1.

Palatable medication (i.e., syrups, throat lozenges, chewable pills) containing even a very small amount of *Chametz*	Forbidden
Palatable medication (i.e., syrups, throat lozenges, chewable pills) that contain *Kitniyot* but not *Chametz*	Permitted
Pills & capsules (that one swallows)	Permitted

If one does not know for certain if there is *Chametz* mixed into a pill, we can rely on the fact that today the vast majority of medical pills do not have *Chametz* mixed in (and in those that do, the *Chametz* is not considered fit for human consumption) and can thus be taken on Passover even by one who is ill to a lesser degree.

Sefirat HaOmer

1. Although one must count the *Omer* every single night in order to be permitted to do so with the blessing, even if one knows that they will be having surgery, or for some reason will not be able to count every day of the *Omer*, they should still begin counting the *Omer* for as long as they are able to with a blessing, and then if they miss some days, continue counting without making the blessing.[479]

H. Fast Days (other than *Tisha B'Av* & *Yom Kippur*)

There are four annual "minor" fast days on which traditionally observant Jews refrain from eating or drinking from dawn until nightfall that same day. In addition to these days, some Jews fast on other specific days throughout the year, such as the day before Passover, "*Ta'anit B'chorot.*"

1a. A sick person in the category of non-life-threatening serious illness [see **pg. 16**, for an explanation of this concept] should not fast on the Fast of *Gedalyah*, Tenth of *Tevet*, or the Seventeenth of *Tammuz*, even if they wish to fast.[480]

1b. There is room for those who are not well to be even more lenient with regard to fasting on *Taanit Esther* than on the above three fast days.[481]

2. A woman who is pregnant or nursing is also not obligated to fast on these days, particularly if the fast distresses her. If fasting distresses her a great deal it is forbidden for her to fast. However, only enough food should be eaten to ensure the well-being of the pregnant woman or the nursing mother and her child, rather than a hearty meal.[482]

---

[479] *Lev Avraham* 20:16 based on *Halichot Shlomo, Moadim* 11:9. In a case of urgent need, one may count the *Omer* after one recites *Maariv*, after *Plag Hamincha.*
[480] *Mishnah Berurah* 550:4.
[481] *Shulchan Aruch OH* 686:2, *Rema.*
[482] *Shulchan Aruch OH* 554:5; *Mishnah Berurah* 550:5; *Shaar Hatziyun* 550:3; *Lev Avraham* 21:5.

3.   A healthy person who is fasting and suffers pain, such as a headache, may take pain-relief pills without water as long as there is not a good flavor associated with the medication. If it does have flavor, it may only be taken in capsule form (or wrapped in thin paper).[483]

I. *Tisha B'Av*

Tisha B'av is a fast of more than 24 hours, commemorating the destruction of the Temple in Jerusalem. The three weeks leading up to *Tisha B'av* begin this season of mourning, which intensifies nine days before the fast, and even more during the week of the fast, culminating in this day of solemnity, prayer, and various ritual observances.

1a. Although it is customary to refrain from hot baths during the nine days prior to *Tisha B'av*, a pregnant woman or anyone who is ill may take a hot bath during this time if it gives relief or comfort,[484] though this should not be done on *Tisha B'av* itself.[485]

1b. Although it is customary to abstain from eating meat or drinking wine during the week or nine days leading up to *Tisha B'av* (with the exclusion of Shabbat),[486] a patient suffering from even a minor illness [see **pg. 16**, for an explanation of this concept], is permitted meat and wine if necessary.[487]

1c. One who must eat animal protein during these days should choose poultry over red meat, unless such meat is more advisable for health reasons, in which case it should be eaten.[488]

1d. One who must have a surgery or procedure during this time period may do so, unless it is elective and can wait, in which case it should be postponed until after *Tisha B'av*.[489]

2a. One who is suffering minor discomfort must still fast.[490] However, one who is sick (bedridden), even with a non-life-threatening illness [see **pg. 16**, for an explanation of this concept], need not fast on *Tisha B'av* and may eat what is necessary in their normal manner.[491] However, one who is healthy but has reason to fear that fasting will lead to illness, should eat only in measurements (see chapter on *Yom Kippur*, "Eating in 'Measurements'").[492]

---

[483] *Lev Avraham* 21:8.
[484] *Mishnah Berurah* 551:88.
[485] Ibid., *Shaar Hatziyun* 94.
[486] *Shulchan Aruch OH* 551:9, though *Sefardim* begin these prohibitions only on *Rosh Chodesh Av*.
[487] *Mishnah Berurah* 551:61, though rarely would wine be necessary.
[488] *Mishnah Berurah* 551:64.
[489] *Torat Hayoledet* 308.
[490] *Aruch Hashulchan OH* 554:7.
[491] *Shulchan Aruch OH* 554:11.
[492] *Lev Avraham* 22:4 in the name of Rav Shlomo Zalman Auerbach.

2b. One who only needs to drink but can avoid eating, for example to prevent a kidney stone, should drink something but not eat. If they must drink normal amounts they may do so; otherwise, they should drink only in measurements.[493]

2c. One who needs to eat should try to eat later than usual so that they fast for at least some time, unless it would be dangerous for them to do so.[494] One who must eat should also consume only the amount needed for their physical well-being.[495]

3. One who has been ill and has now recovered, but is still very weak and in great pain and there is concern that their illness will return, should eat as they regularly do, but should at least avoid eating sweets.[496]

4. One who is experiencing difficulty with their retina, such that dehydration resulting from fasting could lead to loss of vision, even though this is not life-threatening, may drink as their doctor advises (but not eat).[497]

5a. One who is healthy and is fasting, but would like to take a pill to relieve pain, such as from a headache, may take a pill without water, as long as it does not have a good flavor. However, one may not take a pill if they have enjoyment from it in their mouth or throat.[498]

5b. One who is a "Choleh She'ain Bo Sakana," (non-life-threatening serious illness) [see **pg. 16**, for an explanation of this concept], whose doctor orders them to continue taking their medication on Tisha B'av, but is not able to swallow it without water, may take some water (the smallest quantity necessary) to help them swallow the pill.[499] Alternatively, one may follow the guidelines in the chapter on Yom Kippur, section titled, "Taking Medication on Yom Kippur" # 1.

i. Pregnancy and Childbirth

1a. A pregnant woman who feels well should fast on Tisha B'av regardless of which month of pregnancy she is in.[500]

1b. However, if she does not feel well, or did not feel well at the beginning of her pregnancy, she should not fast.[501]

1c. A pregnant woman who feels well, but is weak and is afraid that she will become ill as a result of fasting, should eat in measurements (see chapter on Yom Kippur, "Eating in 'Measurements'").[502]

2. A woman who is nursing and is afraid that she won't produce sufficient milk as a result of fasting, and the baby does not drink formula, should drink normal

---

493 Ibid.
494 Shulchan Aruch OH 554:6 Rema & Mishnah Berurah 13-15.
495 Chayei Adam 135:2.
496 Lev Avraham 22:5.
497 Ibid., 22:3.
498 Ibid., 22:6.
499 Ibid.
500 Shulchan Aruch OH 554:5; Rema 550:1; Lev Avraham 22:2.
501 Mishnah Berurah 554:3 & Shaar Hatziyun 2.
502 Lev Avraham 22:2, in the name of Rav Shlomo Zalman Auerbach.

amounts of fluids, unless she can produce enough milk by drinking only in measurements (see chapter on *Yom Kippur*, "Eating in 'Measurements'").[503]

3. One who has just given birth is not obligated to fast within thirty days of the birth, and should not fast during the first seven days, even if she feels capable.[504] One who miscarried after forty days since conception has the same ruling as a woman who has recently given birth.[505]

---

[503] Ibid.
[504] *Mishnah Berurah* 554:13.
[505] *Lev Avraham* 22:2.

IV. Laws Related to Food & Meals

A. Washing One's Hands Prior to a Meal

This symbolizes the removal of defilement and impurity, and the restoration of spiritual cleanliness and preparation. It is also a reminder of the ancient Temple service in which the "*Kohen*" was required to wash his hands before eating from the separations of food that was set aside for them.

1. If one of a person's hands is partially bandaged, one should wash however much of their hand they are able to and recite the blessing of "*Al Netilat Yadayim.*" Similarly, if one entire hand is unable or not allowed to become wet, one may wash only the other hand and still recite the blessing of "*Al Netilat Yadayim.*"[506] In such a case, the hand that is not washed should be covered with a glove or a cloth so that it does not directly touch any food during the meal.[507]

2a. If one is unable to wash their own hands, anyone is permitted to pour the water over their hands for them.[508]

2b. If a patient is fed bread by an attendant, it is the patient and not the attendant whose hands should be washed, even though the patient does not handle the bread.[509] If the patient has no hands and thus does not touch the bread, then he or she does not need to wash at all.

3. If one is unable to pour water on their hands and has no one to do it for them, it is not sufficient to simply place one's hands under a faucet without using a utensil. Thus, in such a case, one may only eat bread if they are wearing a glove or a cloth on their hands when they touch it.[510]

4. One is generally not permitted to perform religious activities in a restroom, including washing their hands before prayer or eating bread (although there is more room for leniency in the case of washing hands before prayer).[511] However, if one has nowhere else to wash their hands, some authorities permit washing them in the restroom, provided they dry them and make the blessing outside of the restroom.[512]

---

[506] *Shulchan Aruch OH* 162:10 & *Mishnah Berurah* 68; *Yechaveh Daat* 2:19; *Lev Avraham* 8:1.
[507] *Mishnah Berurah* 162:69; *Lev Avraham* 8:1.
[508] *Shulchan Aruch OH* 159:11.
[509] Ibid., 163:2; *Nishmat Avraham OH* 163:2 (2).
[510] *Lev Avraham* 8:4.
[511] *Igrot Moshe EH* 1:114.
[512] *Minchat Yitzchak* 1:60; *Yechaveh Daat* 3:1.

B. Blessings

1a.   If one takes a drink of water because they were instructed to do so by their doctor or in order to swallow pills, but not because of thirst, they do not make a blessing before or after.[513]

1b.   If one drinks water in order to swallow a pill, but then becomes thirsty and drinks more water, they would need to make a blessing beforehand, and afterwards if they drink enough water to become obligated to recite the blessing after consuming liquids (about 3 ounces) after they became thirsty.[514]

1c.   If one takes medicine with a liquid that has a good flavor, or any beverage other than water, they must make the appropriate blessings before and after, even though they only drank the liquid for medicinal purposes (i.e., to help them swallow a pill) because they have some enjoyment from the taste.[515]

1d.   One who has to eat non-kosher food in order to save their life should still recite a blessing of *Shehakol* before eating the food because since they needed to eat it, the food is permitted and they are doing the Mitzvah of saving their life.[516]

2.   One who is not fed through their mouth, but by something like an NG tube or a PEG, does not make a blessing before or after they are fed because it is not considered "eating."[517]

3.   If there is a foul odor in the room such that one cannot make a blessing, they may have the blessing in mind and then eat or drink.[518]

C. Medication

1a.   A patient who is not seriously ill may swallow medication unfit for consumption as human food, i.e., pills, even if derived from non-kosher ingredients if this is required for their healing. If possible, it is preferred that one find a kosher alternative (there are many Israeli-produced medicines that are certified kosher).[519]

1b.   It is preferable to take a non-kosher medicine in pill form, rather than as a pleasant-tasting medicine such as chewable tablets.[520] One should not take

---

[513] *Shulchan Aruch OH* 204:7; *Lev Avraham* 10:3.

[514] *Lev Avraham*, Ibid.

[515] *Shulchan Aruch OH* 204:8 & *Mishnah Berurah* 43. The *Shaar Hatziyun* 37 explains that this is true even if the flavor is not very good, as long as it palatable; *Lev Avraham* 10:2-3.

[516] *Shulchan Aruch OH* 196:2; *Mishnah Berurah* 196:5; *Nishmat Avraham OH* 196:1.

[517] *Lev Avraham* 10:7 based on *Minchat Chinuch* 313:2 and others.

[518] *Torat Hayoledet* pg. 427; *Mishnah Berurah* 62:8.

[519] *Lev Avraham* 12:2-3; *Shulchan Aruch YD* 155:3. Exceptions to this ruling include meat cooked with dairy products and actual *Chametz* during Passover unless such products are needed as a life-saving measure.

[520] See *Minchat Shlomo* 1:17, where Rav Shlomo Zalman Auerbach rules that swallowing medicine pills does not constitute an act of eating because they are made to be swallowed and are intended only for sick individuals, and thus swallowing them is regarded as abnormal benefit and is permissible even for a patient who is not seriously ill. Furthermore, Rav Waldenburg notes that medications are generally only a rabbinic prohibition because they are taken in such small doses (*Tzitz Eliezer* 6:16).

pleasant-tasting liquid medications containing non-kosher ingredients unless they are dangerously ill, in which case all instructions given by the doctor should be carefully followed, including taking the medication for the prescribed number of days, even though the symptoms may have subsided, unless an equally effective kosher medicine is readily available. There is additional room for leniency when it comes to allowing children to take pleasant-tasting medicines.[521]

D. Meat & Milk

1. Although it is the generally accepted custom to wait six hours before eating dairy products after eating meat, a non-seriously ill patient, a woman within thirty days of childbirth, a pregnant woman suffering discomfort because of her pregnancy, or a nursing mother with insufficient milk, may wait only one hour after eating meat if necessary. However, they should make sure to recite the appropriate blessing after eating the meat meal and rinse their mouth out before proceeding to eat dairy products.[522]

2. One who takes a pill made of meat products, such as liver extract, does not need to wait six hours before eating dairy.[523]

---

[521] Rabbi Dovid Heber, "A Kashrus Guide to Medications, Vitamins, and Nutritional Supplements" (based on rulings of Rabbi Moshe Heinemann) Star-K Kashrus Kurrents, http://www.star-k.org/kashrus/kk-medi-guide.htm#fA. ; See also Mesorah 7:91-96 & 14:93.

[522] Lev Avraham 12:5.

[523] Igrot Moshe YD 2:26.

V. Prayer

Traditionally observant Jews pray three times a day and also recite a number of other prayers at various times, such as after a meal. These prayers are usually said quietly, moving one's lips but without speaking loudly enough for others to hear. While praying, one refrains from any interruptions, even if someone else tries to get one's attention.

1. Although one is supposed to wash one's hands after sleep and before prayer, if one is unable to get to water or have it brought to their bed, one should instead thoroughly wipe one's hands on a cloth or garment and then say the blessing, "*Al Netillat Yadayim*."[524] If water becomes available later, they should then wash their hands but not say the blessing again.

2a. Although one who is healthy is not supposed to eat or drink anything (other than water, tea, or coffee) before saying the morning prayers,[525] one who is ill may do so.[526] However, if possible, even someone who is ill should at least say the morning blessings and the first paragraph of the *Shema* before eating anything.[527]

2b. On Shabbat and major festivals one must also hear *Kiddush* before eating.[528] However, one who is weak may eat as much as they need to strengthen themselves before praying or reciting *Kiddush*.[529]

3a. A patient who is unable to speak should still pray through thoughts alone, without words, if that is possible.[530]

3b. One who is too weak to pray can also listen to another person say the prayers and respond "Amen" to the blessings.[531]

4. One who is too weak to say all of the prayers is exempt from praying, but should at least say the morning blessings and the *Shema*, or at least its first verse.[532] One who is able to pray a little bit more, but not the entire standard *Shemoneh Esreh* prayer, should instead say the "*Havinenu*" substitute for the middle thirteen blessings.[533]

5a. Although one is normally supposed to stand while reciting the *Shemoneh Esreh* prayer without leaning on anything,[534] if one is unable to stand but can

---

[524] *Mishnah Berurah* 1:2, 4:16, 92:21.

[525] *Shulchan Aruch OH* 89:3 & *Mishnah Berurah* 21-22.

[526] Ibid., 89:4. Since the prohibition against eating or drinking before prayer is because it is seen as conceited to prioritize ones physical desires before God, it follows that when the purpose of eating is for the sake of healing, it does not seem conceited, and is thus permitted even for one who is not completely sick (*Mishnah Berurah* 89:24).

[527] Ibid., 89:3; *Lev Avraham* 5:15. If it is difficult to say both the morning blessings and the *"Shema"* before eating, one can just say the *"Shema"* (*Mishnah Berurah* 99:22).

[528] *Lev Avraham* 5:15; *Mishnah Berurah* 286:9. *Beur Halachah* 289 s.v. *Chovat Kiddush*.

[529] *Mishnah Berurah* 286:9. See also *Shaar Hatziyun* 9 that one may certainly eat if necessary before *Mussaf*.

[530] *Shulchan Aruch OH* 94:6 *Rema*; *Mishnah Berurah* 62:6.

[531] *Shulchan Aruch OH* 594:1 *Rema*.

[532] *Mishnah Berurah* 94:21; *Lev Avraham* 5:30.

[533] *Shulchan Aruch OH* 110:1.

[534] Ibid., 94:8.

concentrate while leaning on something, they may do so.[535] One who is unable to stand, even while leaning for support, may recite the *Shemoneh Esreh* while seated.[536] If unable to sit, one may recite it reclining,[537] preferably with their head and shoulders elevated.[538] If this is not possible either, one should lie on their side, even if just slightly.[539] If even this is impossible, one may pray while lying flat on one's back.[540]

5b. A patient who could stand, but is able to pray better while seated or lying down, may do so, but should try to stand during the times that one bows during the *Shemoneh Esreh*.[541]

6. One who recites the *Shemoneh Esreh* prayer while seated in a wheelchair should ideally move it backwards (or ask someone to move it) the distance of three steps at the conclusion of the *Shemoneh Esreh*, as they would when reciting it while standing.[542]

7a. When praying, one should see oneself as standing with a sense of trepidation before a King. One should therefore not wear only pajamas if possible, and should have their entire body covered while praying.[543]

7b. A man should not pray in only a hospital gown, but must also have a physical separation such as a bathrobe belt or underwear at the waist.[544]

8. Although one who is in the midst of reciting the *Shemoneh Esreh* prayer is not permitted to interrupt it in any manner, one who has any urgent medical condition during prayer may interrupt their prayers to address the condition, and may then continue in their prayers from the point at which they interrupted. [545]

Earliest time for Prayer, *Tallit*, *Tefillin*

9. The earliest time that one may recite the blessing for putting on his *Tallit* and *Tefillin* is when there is enough daylight to allow one to recognize an acquaintance from a distance of four "*Amot*" (about seven feet)[546] and can distinguish between sky-blue and white.[547] This time is referred to as "*Mi'sheyakir*." The exact time depends on a number of factors, such as location and season, but is generally accepted as approximately 50 minutes before sunrise.[548]

---

535 *Mishnah Berurah* 94:24.
536 Ibid.
537 *Shulchan Aruch OH* 94:6; *Mishnah Berurah* 94:20.
538 *Nishmat Avraham* 63:1.
539 *Shulchan Aruch OH* 94:6; *Shulchan Aruch OH* 63:1; *Mishnah Berurah* 63:2 & 4; *Nishmat Avraham OH* 63:1.
540 *Aruch Hashulchan OH* 63:5.
541 *Guide for the Jewish Hospital Patient* 14.
542 *Lev Avraham* 5:20.
543 *Mishnah Berurah* 91:1,2,11.
544 *Shulchan Aruch OH* 91:2; *Mishnah Berurah* 91:5.
545 *Lev Avraham* 5:26 in the name of Rav Eliyashiv. This includes stopping to eat and make the appropriate blessing if one is having a hypoglycemic attack (sudden onset of low blood sugar levels).
546 *Igrot Moshe OH* 1:136.
547 *Shulchan Aruch OH* 18:3.
548 *Ezras Torah Luach*; *Guide to Halachos*, 126. Rav Henkin rules that in a case of need one may pray and put on *Tallit* and *Tefillin* 72 minutes before the time of sunrise.

10. Although the *Shema* and its blessings should also be said after "*Mi'sheyakir*," if one is unable to wait until then, they may be said as early as dawn ("*Alot Hashachar*"),[549] which is about 72 minutes before sunrise,[550] but the exact time can vary throughout the year.

11. The *Shemoneh Esreh* is ideally said at sunrise, but in a case of need may also be said as early as dawn ("*Alot Hashachar*").[551]

12. A patient who must pray early, such as one who is having a surgery early in the morning and will not be able to pray or put on *Tallit* or *Tefillin* that day following the procedure, may begin praying after dawn ("*Alot Hashachar*") up until the blessing of "*Yotzer Or*" in the first blessing of the *Shema*, and once they have reached the time of "*Mi'sheyakir*" may put on their *Tallit* (and *Tefillin* if it is not Shabbat), make the appropriate blessings and continue with their prayers.[552] If this is also not possible, one may put on their *Tallit* and *Tefillin* (without the blessings) and say all of the morning prayers as early as "*Alot Hashachar*."[553] If even this is not possible, and one would like to say some prayers with their *Tallit* and *Tefillin* on even before "*Alot Hashachar*," they may do so, but may not recite their blessings when putting them on, and may only say the morning prayers after "*Alot Hashachar*."[554]

Prayer in an unclean environment

13. One is not permitted to pray or study Torah in the immediate presence of feces or urine, unless it is covered (for this purpose, even a see-through plastic receptacle may serve as a cover)[555] and no foul odor is present.[556]

14. A patient who is in a place where it is not permitted to pray because of a foul odor, and who is unable to leave that room, may not pray or even think the prayers,[557] but should think to themselves that they would like to pray if they could, but are not allowed to.[558] If the room becomes clean while there is still time in the day, one should then say their prayers.

15. A patient with a catheter in their bladder through which urine passes into a bag may pray and study Torah provided that there is no foul odor emanating from it.[559]

16. A patient with an ileostomy or colostomy, by which an opening is created to provide an alternative channel for feces to leave their body, may continue to pray and study Torah as they normally would, as long as the opening is covered and does not omit

---

549 *Shulchan Aruch OH* 58:1 & 58:3.
550 *Beur Halachah* 89:1 s.v. "*V'em Hitpalel*."
551 *Shulchan Aruch OH* 89:1 & 8.
552 Ibid., 58:3; *Mishnah Berurah* 58:13; *Beur Halachah* 58 s.v. "*Zman*."
553 *Nishmat Avraham OH* 58:1 (based on *Mishnah Berurah* 58:16).
554 Ibid. Another option is to put on *Tallit* and *Tefillin* early, without a blessing, but to move around the *Tallit* and wiggle the *Tefillin* at *Mi'sheyakir*, and then recite the blessing over both of them at that time.
555 *Shulchan Aruch OH* 76:1.
556 Ibid., 77:1 & *Mishnah Berurah* 2; *Mishnah Berurah* 79:2, *Beur Halachah* s.v. "*Tzoah*"; *Shulchan Aruch OH* 76:1; *Shulchan Aruch OH* 87:3.
557 *Shulchan Aruch OH* 62:4 Rema.
558 *Mishnah Berurah* 62:9; *Beur Halachah* 76:8 s.v. "*Tzarich*."
559 *Lev Avraham* 5:25.

a foul odor. One should clean and cover the site before beginning to pray or study Torah.[560]

17. One should be very careful to respect the holiness of sacred books. Therefore, if one is going to relieve themselves by their bedside, for example, and they have holy books beside their bed, they should cover the books. However, if the table is four by four "*Tefachim*" (a "*Tefach*" is about 3.5 inches) and has solid sides (rather than legs) that are at least ten "*Tefachim*" high, one need not be concerned about covering the books since they are located in a different and distinct space from a *Halachic* perspective.[561]

A. *Tefillin*

Tefillin (phylacteries) are black boxes worn on the arm and head of male worshippers during weekday morning prayers. These boxes contain writings from the Torah, are considered holy and should be treated with utmost care.

1. The *Mitzvah* of *Tefillin* consists of two separate commandments, one pertaining to the one worn on the arm (referred to herein as "*Tefillin* of the hand"), and the other, to the one worn on the head ("*Tefillin* of the head"). Therefore, one who is unable to put on both, must still put on whichever one he can.[562]

2a. If one is right-handed or ambidextrous, *Tefillin* are placed on the left arm. If a right-handed man puts his *Tefillin* on his right arm, he has not fulfilled the *Mitzvah* of putting on *Tefillin*.[563] One who is left-handed puts his *Tefillin* on his right arm.[564] Thus, throughout this chapter whenever we refer to the left arm, we mean whichever arm is not dominant.

2b. Although *Tefillin* of the hand should be placed over the lower half of the biceps, one who is unable to place *Tefillin* on that part of his arm may place it over the upper half of the bicep and make the blessing.[565]

2c. One who does not have a forearm from the elbow downward should nevertheless put on the *Tefillin* of the hand.[566] When one then puts on their *Tefillin* of the head, they should make both blessings and have the *Tefillin* of the hand in mind as well.[567]

2d. One who has most of his arm, but no hand, still puts *Tefillin* on that arm and says the blessing in the normal manner.[568]

---

[560] Ibid., 5:26.
[561] Ibid., 6:12.
[562] *Shulchan Aruch OH* 26:1.
[563] *Mishnah Berurah* 27:1.
[564] *Shuhlchan Aruch OH* 27:6.
[565] Ibid., 27:1 & *Mishnah Berurah* 4.
[566] Ibid., 27:1 *Rema*.
[567] *Beur Halacha* 27:1 s.v. "*B'lo Bracha.*"
[568] *Mishnah Berurah* 27:5.

2e.   One whose arm is missing the entire part of the upper arm bone usually covered by the biceps should not put his hand *Tefillin* on any stump that remains on his left arm. Such a person would be exempt from putting on the *Tefillin* of the hand, but may put *Tefillin* on his right arm without reciting the blessing.[569]

2f.   One who must put *Tefillin* on his right arm generally does not make the blessing if he puts them on his left arm. However, since *Ashkenazim* recite two blessings on *Tefillin*, they should recite both of the blessings on the head *Tefillin*, with the intention that the blessing "*Lehaniach Tefillin*" applies to the *Tefillin* of the hand as well.[570]

3.   One for whom it is very painful to put *Tefillin* on his arm is exempt from putting on the *Tefillin* of the hand (even if there is room on the arm to do so), and should thus put on only the *Tefillin* of the head.[571]

4a.   One who puts on only *Tefillin* of the head and not the arm should:

- If he is *Sephardi*, recite only the blessing of "*Al Mitzvat Tefillin*."
- If he is *Ashkenazi*, recite both "*Lehaniach Tefillin*" and "*Al Mitzvat Tefillin*."[572]

4b.   One who puts on only *Tefillin* of the arm, and not the head, should recite only the blessing of "*Lehaniach Tefillin*" according to both *Sephardi* and *Ashkenazi* practice.[573]

5.   One whose middle finger of the left hand has been amputated should wind the strap around his index finger instead.[574]

6a.   Nothing should be between one's body and the *Tefillin*. One whose IV tubes make it impossible to wind *Tefillin* around his arm seven times as he normally does, should still put *Tefillin* on his left arm, but should simply strap the box to his bicep and then draw the strap directly down to his middle finger, without winding it around his forearm. The blessing is nevertheless made when putting *Tefillin* on in this manner, even if it is strapped only to the bicep, and not to any of one's forearm or finger.[575]

6b.   A person whose left arm is in a plaster cast should still put *Tefillin* on that arm and not their right arm. As long as the box of the *Tefillin* is in contact with his skin, even if the straps are wrapped around the cast, he may make the blessing over fulfilling the *Mitzvah* of *Tefillin* in this manner.[576] However, if the box itself is on the cast and not directly touching his skin, he may recite only the blessing for the *Tefillin* of the head.[577]

[569] Ibid., 27:6.
[570] *Beur Halachah* 27:1 s.v. "*B'lo Bracha.*"
[571] *Mishnah Berurah* 27:29.
[572] *Shulchan Aruch OH 26:2 Rema; Beur Halacha* 27:1 s.v. "*B'lo.*"
[573] *Shulchan Aruch OH 26:2 Rema.*
[574] *Lev Avraham* 4:5.
[575] Ibid., 4:4.
[576] Ibid., 4:3; *Mishnah Berurah* 27:16, 18.
[577] Ibid.

6c. If a cast, bandage, or the like covers the entire area designated for the hand *Tefillin*, the *Tefillin* can be placed on top of it,[578] but without reciting the blessing. However, since *Ashkenazim* recite two blessings on *Tefillin*, they should recite both of the blessings on the head *Tefillin*, with the intention that the blessing "*Lehaniach Tefillin*" applies to the *Tefillin* of the hand as well.[579] *Sephardim* just make the blessing of "*Al Mitzvat Tefillin*" on their head *Tefillin*. When the hand *Tefillin* is worn in this manner, it should be covered by a shirt, jacket or other garment, but it may never be worn over a shirt or other garment.[580]

7. If one's left arm is paralyzed,[581] or has hand atrophy, he should still put *Tefillin* on that arm.[582] However, if in addition to suffering paralysis, the arm has completely lost all sensation, it is considered not to exist for these purposes and he should put *Tefillin* on his other arm.[583]

8. If both arms are paralyzed, he should have *Tefillin* put on his left arm for him by someone else,[584] and recite the blessings as he normally does.[585]

9. If there is no man available to assist one in putting on *Tefillin*, he may allow a woman to put them on him, and he may make the blessing.[586]

10. One whose head is bandaged should still put on his head *Tefillin*. If he is *Sephardi*, a blessing is not made on the head *Tefillin*. An *Ashkenazi* would make the blessing, "*Al Mitzvat Tefillin*" in such a case only if the box of the *Tefillin* lies in direct contact with the head, even if the straps are on top of the bandage. However, if the box lies on the bandage, he does not recite the blessing.[587]

11. One suffering from an illness should put *Tefillin* on only if he is able to concentrate on the *Mitzvah*.[588] While wearing *Tefillin* he must also maintain a clean body.[589] If he is suffering from severe diarrhea, or flatulence that makes him unable to avoid passing gas, he may not put *Tefillin* on.[590]

12. It is forbidden to sleep, or even take a nap, while wearing *Tefillin*.[591]

---

[578] *Mishnah Berurah* 27:18.
[579] *Beur Halachah* 27:1 s.v. "*B'lo.*"
[580] *Mishnah Berurah* 27:16.
[581] *Igrot Moshe OH* 1:8-9.
[582] *Lev Avraham* 4:7.
[583] Ibid., 4:8; *Nishmat Avraham EH* 169:5.
[584] *Mishnah Berurah* 27:6,22.
[585] *Lev Avraham* 4:9.
[586] Ibid., 4:10.
[587] *Mishnah Berurah* 27:16.
[588] *Shulchan Aruch OH* 38:1 *Rema*.
[589] *Mishnah Berurah* 38:2.
[590] *Shulchan Aruch OH* 38:1.
[591] Ibid., 44:1. The *Shulchan Aruch* there suggests that one who can't avoid momentary sleep while wearing *Tefillin* should put a cloth over their *Tefillin*. If one is unable to avoid dozing off while wearing *Tefillin*, they should consult a rabbinic authority for guidance.

VI. Interactions with Individuals of the Opposite Gender

Judaism generally prohibits a man and a woman who are not immediate relatives from being alone together, or any sort of sexual physical contact. Caregivers should be cognizant of these sensitivities and avoid isolation or physical contact with a traditionally observant Jewish patient or arrange for a caregiver of the same gender if possible. These rules were established to promote modesty and appropriate behavior, and to prevent any chance of improper conduct or accusations of such. These rules should not be misinterpreted as an inference of superiority or inferiority between the sexes. In professional and medical situations, there are occasionally some exceptions to these rules, as discussed below.

A. Seclusion ("*Yichud*")

1a.   Although it is forbidden for people of the opposite gender to be secluded together, a patient may be in the room with their doctor or nurse of the opposite gender if the door remains unlocked and it is possible, and indeed not unlikely, that another person may enter at any time.[592]

1b.   Some permit such seclusion even if the door is locked, as long as there are people around with the key who can easily enter at any moment.[593]

1c.   In all cases it is best to avoid being in private with an individual of the opposite gender and it is preferable that another reliable person, such as a nurse or member of the patient's family, be present in the room when possible.[594]

2a.   A married woman may travel alone in an ambulance with a male driver, even at night within the city, assuming her husband is in that city. However, if they are traveling outside of the city, or the woman is single, they may do so only if it is possible to see into the ambulance through its windows.[595]

2b.   If the patient is seriously ill, they may travel in an ambulance even in violation of the laws of seclusion.[596]

2c.   If a person is afraid to travel in the ambulance alone or wants to avoid violating the prohibition against seclusion, someone else may travel in the ambulance with them, even on Shabbat and even if the driver is Jewish.[597]

---

[592]   *Lev Avraham* 49:4 quoting *Teshuvot HaRashba* 1:1251, *Teshuvot HaRadvaz* 1:121, R, Yona *Sefer HaYirah* 234-237, *Tzitz Eliezer* 6:40 (23).
[593]   Ibid., 49:4 quoting *Tzitz Eliezer* 6:40 (12:10),
[594]   Ibid., 34:32.
[595]   Ibid., 49:7; *Nishmat Avraham EH* 22:8 & 4a.
[596]   Ibid., 49:8; *Nishmat Avraham EH* 22:1 & OH 278:1 (34).
[597]   Ibid., 49:8 in the name of Rav Shlomo Zalman Auerbach. This leniency applies primarily if the goal is to calm the fears of a dangerously ill patient, but not if it is <u>only</u> to avoid violating the laws of seclusion, since those restrictions are waived for a dangerously ill patient. Another Jew should thus not ride in the ambulance on Shabbat just for that

3.   It is permitted to visit an individual of the opposite gender in the hospital, but one should be cognizant of modesty and avoid being secluded in the room with the patient.[598]

B. Physical Contact

1.   Jewish Law generally prohibits a man and a woman from any physical contact, including shaking hands, even if one of the people is ill.[599]

2.   However, physicians or nurses are permitted to make physical contact with a patient of the opposite gender in the course of medical examinations if necessary.[600]

3.   Another exception occurs when a person is very fearful: an individual of the opposite gender may then hold one's hand or touch their head in order to calm or strengthen their spirit. In such a situation, it would be best to touch clothing or use a glove in order to avoid touching the person's skin directly.[601]

4.   More restrictions are placed on treating patients with gastro-intestinal or gynecological issues, particularly with men treating women in such situations, out of fear that indecency might occur when a man must clean a woman or help her to the bathroom, thus coming into constant bodily contact.[602] Each situation is unique, and one should consult a rabbi to discuss the specifics.

---

purpose (*Nishmat Avraham EH* 22:1 (4), pg. 207).

[598] Ibid., 31:2 based on *Aruch Hashulchan YD* 335:11.

[599] Ibid., 34:4.

[600] *Nishmat Avraham YD* 195:17 (11) quoting the *Shach YD* 195:20.

[601] Ibid., in the name of Rav Yehoshua Neuwirth. For an in-depth discussion of the effectiveness of wearing gloves to mitigate the prohibition in such circumstances, see Rav Ovadia Yosef's *Taharat Habayit* vol. 2, pgs. 208-214.

[602] *Shulchan Aruch YD* 335:10; *Nishmat Avraham YD* 335:24-25; *Nishmat Avraham EH* 22:5 (*Rema*).

VII. *Kohanim*[603]

A *Kohen* (male of "priestly" descent) is bound by the verse in the Torah which states, "Speak to the *Kohanim*, the sons of Aharon and tell them each of you shall not contaminate himself to a dead person among his people" (Leviticus 21:1), which prohibits him from being in situations that cause him to be "contaminated" by ritual impurity. This ritual impurity is imparted via proximity to a corpse or a body part, and may affect him as a patient, physician, hospital employee, or visitor to the hospital.

1. A *Kohen* may not be in a room or area containing a corpse or part of one, or a severed limb of a living person.[604] This prohibition also applies to all rooms, corridors, or staircases through which the corpse will be transported.

2. When a deceased patient is in a room, the entire intended path of egress is forbidden to a *Kohen*. This includes:

   • The entire hallway from the room to the elevator (even the part of the hallway that will not be traversed, until the hallway ends at a wall or a door).

   • The elevator itself.

   • The hallway from the elevator to the morgue, or in the case of direct removal by the mortuary, the loading dock.

   • The hallway from the morgue to the loading dock.

3a. A *Kohen* who is not seriously ill may thus not enter a hospital when it is known that a corpse is in the building. However, when there is a need to enter the hospital, we rely on the ruling that where a majority of corpses will be deceased Gentiles (who are not subject to the Torah's system of purity and impurity), we are lenient to enable the performance of a *Mitzvah*,[605] and certainly in order to seek medical treatment.[606]

3b. Outside of Israel, a *Kohen* may visit a close relative in the hospital since we assume that the majority of patients are not Jewish.[607]

4a. A *Kohen* who is a patient, or visiting someone in the hospital, must be especially careful on a unit or floor that frequently treats dying patients, and take the following precautions:[608]

   a) Make certain that there are no decedents on the floor before entering.

   b) Keep the door to the patient's room closed unless it must be opened for a specific need.

   c) Once again verify that no one has died before opening the door to leave the room.

---

[603] The status of hospitals can vary based on the location of their morgue, structure of their facility and percentage of Jewish patients. One should contact a knowledgeable local Rav or Jewish chaplain to determine the accessibility of their hospital for Kohanim.

[604] *Shulchan Aruch YD* 369, 371:1

[605] *Shach YD* 372:2.

[606] *Lev Avraham* 41:6; *Igrot Moshe YD* 1:230:3

[607] *Igrot Moshe YD* 2:166. In addition to close relatives, Reb Moshe extends this permission to visiting a non-relative if family tension will occur as a result of the *Kohen* not visiting.

[608] *Lev Avraham* 41:8.

4b.   A *Kohen* who learns that someone on the floor where he is a patient or a visitor has died must remain in the room that he is in and close the doors until the corpse has been removed.[609]

4c.   A *Kohen* who is not in a room when he finds out about a corpse in the area must leave immediately if possible, and expedite his exit by taking the most direct and quickest route possible in order to limit his exposure to possible ritual contamination.

---

[609]   *Nishmat Avraham YD* 372:1.

VIII. Death and Post-Mortem Care[610]

A. The Actively Dying Patient

1. When it seems that the patient may have begun the active dying process, one should consult a rabbi, chaplain, or doctor who is knowledgeable in these matters, to determine if the patient may have entered the status of *"Gosses,"* which means a person who is expected to die shortly. If the patient may be in that category, we must treat them as delicately as possible so as not to hasten their death in any way.

2. One should not move or touch a patient determined to be a *"Gosses"* unless it is for the patient's own good:

    - A physician or anyone else who needs to treat such a patient must do whatever is **medically necessary** until the patient has died, because we do anything to save a life, when necessary.

    - However, if there is nothing medical that can be done for the patient, we must show extreme caution, particularly in a hospital where even many **routine** examinations should be avoided. For example, drawing blood for laboratory tests, checking blood pressure, temperature, and even heartbeat, should not be done if, in any case, the results of these examinations will not affect the medical treatment of the patient.

    - On the other hand, if the patient is alert and will realize that these routine actions have been stopped, and this knowledge and its resultant despair and hopelessness may aggravate the patient's condition, then these treatments should continue, but with the absolute minimum physical contact needed to put the patient at ease.

    - All nursing care that is necessary for the patient's physical and mental comfort, such as washing, cleaning, and changing the bed linen must still be done, even on Shabbat.

    - It is permitted to provide supportive contact, such as stroking the hand of a *Gosses* who is frightened so as to calm him or her.[611]

3a. It is customary to maintain a state of reverence and respect in the presence of a dying patient, and not to speak about mundane matters, unless the patient wants such conversation.[612]

3b. It is also important to avoid loud crying in the presence of a dying patient, while they are still alive, so as not to frighten them.[613]

---

[610] I would like to thank Rabbi Elchonon Zohn, director of the National Association of Chevra Kadisha, who was consulted extensively in the preparation of this section.

[611] All based on *Nishmat Avraham YD* 339 (3 & 6); see also pgs. 318-319 in the English edition. The *Nishmat Avraham* points out that in the emergency room, one may carefully move a *Gosses* when that patient's bed, or one of his or her limbs, is in a position that makes it impossible to move a **seriously ill** patient to where they can receive appropriate treatment (for example, in order to move the **seriously ill** patient to the intensive care unit or to connect them to a respirator). This is permitted because there is a great need to try to save the life of a **seriously ill patient**, in which case one may move the arm of a *Gosses* or his or her bed as long as it is done very carefully and there is only a possibility that his or her death will be hastened by doing so.

[612] *Kol Bo al Aveilut* vol. 1, pg. 22. Some also avoid eating or drinking in the presence of a dying patient.

[613] Ibid.

4.   It is ideal to not allow a person to die alone, if possible.[614]

5.   Anyone in the presence of another person who dies is obligated to ritually tear a portion of their clothing at the moment of death.[615] However, today this is not always practiced:

- People who are **not related** to the deceased, such as hospital staff, generally **do not tear their clothing** at this time[616] because we are concerned that nobody would then want to be at the side of a dying person if they have to tear their clothing at the moment of death.[617] However, anyone in the presence of one who dies should recite the words "*Baruch Dayan Haemet*" (Blessed is the true Judge).[618]

- People who **are closely related** to the deceased frequently **do tear their clothing** (and recite the full "*Dayan Haemet*" blessing) at the moment of death. However, **many are accustomed to wait until the funeral** because that is considered the time of the most intense grief. Furthermore, at the funeral the mourners are more focused, the entire family is gathered together and the rabbi can assist them in tearing their clothing properly.[619]

When Death Occurs

1.   When a death occurs, one should make sure that the death certificate is signed by a physician and that a family member signs a release form (not on Shabbat) so that a mortuary can pick up the deceased.

- Since the release form may not be signed by an observant Jew on Shabbat, it may be signed before Shabbat (even though the patient is still alive) or one may give verbal authorization on Shabbat instead of signing. If the family is unreachable on Shabbat they must wait until after Shabbat to sign it.

2.   One should also notify their rabbi and a Jewish mortuary. Some mortuaries may not respond on Shabbat, though they usually have an operator service

---

[614] *Rema, YD* 339:4. This is because we believe that it is beneficial to the dying person to sense the presence of his or her loved ones during the last moments of life (*Kol Bo al Aveilut* vol. 1, pg. 22 quoting *Maavor Yabok* 5:28). For this reason one may even remain with a dying person if the time for communal prayer will pass (*R. Akivah Eiger YD* 339). It is also important for someone to be with the dying patient so that they can ensure that the proper prayers are said, and that the body of the deceased is in the proper position and thus does not become disgraced (*Divrei Sofrim* 329:4 (28)).

[615] *Shulchan Aruch YD* 340:5; *Igrot Moshe CH"M* 2:73 (9).

[616] *Nishmat Avraham OH* 233:2 (6) & *YD* 340:34(2); *Gesher Hachaim* 4:9. Some say that they should nevertheless tear a small amount at the bottom of their garment (*Minhagim V'Kitzur Piskei Halachot Hanechutzot Al Kol Tzara Shelo Tavo, Chevra Kaddisha Yitav Lev of Satmar* 3; *Divrei Sofrim* 340:29).

[617] Ibid. According to this reasoning, those who would want to be with the dying person regardless of the fact that they will have to tear their clothing, such as a close student of the patient, should indeed tear their clothing if they are present at the moment of death.

[618] *Baer Heiteiv, OH* 223:6.

[619] *Gesher Hachaim* 4:6; *Min HaOlam V'ad HaOlam*, 5:27. As above, perhaps even those who do not tear their garment until the funeral should nevertheless make a small tear at the bottom of their garment when they are present at the moment of death. Furthermore, perhaps family members who are more distant relatives, and will thus not be tearing their clothing at the funeral, should tear their clothing at the moment of the patient's passing if they are present. One should seek competent rabbinic guidance on these questions.

that will take the message and give instructions, and it is often helpful to notify them before Shabbat (especially the mortuary in case one isn't available in the hospital to sign the release, it is often sufficient to have made arrangements with a mortuary).

3. If it has not already been determined, the family will have to decide the **place** of burial and the **timing** of the funeral (taking into consideration both the requirement for prompt burial as well as the importance of properly honoring the deceased by getting the word out and ensuring that loved ones have time to arrive from out of town).

B. Positioning of the Body

1a. After death, a human body is still considered sacred and should be treated with the utmost respect.[620] After death, a nurse generally cleans the body and prepares it to be transfered to the morgue or mortuary. Observant Jews frequently ask that the body be left untouched until the mortuary arrives to handle it in accordance with Jewish custom.

1b. Once death has been established, it is customary not to touch the corpse for about 20 minutes,[621] after which some of the following customs are observed by family members if possible (though if one is too overwhelmed to do this themselves, they may wait for the chaplain, rabbi, or mortuary to assist them):

2. One should open a window in the room if possible.[622]

3a. The eyes and mouth should be gently closed[623] and the head elevated if possible.

3b. If the mouth remains open, then:

- The chin should be tied with a bandage or towel around the head,[624] or

- One may place a prop, such as a rolled up towel, under the chin, or

- If the mouth still remains open, then it should be covered with a clean cloth.[625]

4. The body should be lying on its back, and straightened out as much as possible.[626] This includes:

- Legs straight out.

- Arms straightened at the side of the body.

- Hands are to be opened as completely as possible, with the palms facing the ceiling, if possible.

---

[620] *Gesher Hachaim* vol. 1, 5:1.
[621] Ibid., 3:2 (1). This is because for a short time the patient may still be classified as dying, but not yet fully dead, so we do not want to do anything that would hasten their death.
[622] *Zichron Meir al Aveilut*, 166. There is also a custom when a person dies to pour out all drawn water in the surroundings (*Shulchan Aruch YD* 339:5), but this is not practiced in a hospital (*Nishmat Avraham YD* 339:5 (11)).
[623] *Shulchan Aruch YD* 352:4. The *Chochmat Adam* 157:9 mentions a custom of having the firstborn son of the deceased be the one to close the eyes when possible.
[624] Ibid.
[625] *Yesodei Semachot*, pg. 142, 6a.
[626] *Gesher Hachaim* vol. 1, 15:2 (6).

- It is important to ensure that none of the limbs of the deceased hang off the side of the bed or stretcher.

5. If the body must be turned for any reason, it may be turned on either side but not face down.

6a. The body and head should be completely covered with a sheet (not a warm heavy blanket).

6b. When the body is disrobed, the genital area should remain covered by a cloth at all times.

7. The room which the body is in should be kept as cool as possible.[627]

8. When the body is placed on the appropriate stretcher and transferred to the morgue or mortuary, it should always be transported feet first.

C. Treatment of the body on Shabbat and Festivals

1. The book "*Shemirat Shabbat Kehilchatah*" states, "On Shabbat and Yom Tov [Festivals], a corpse is *muktzeh* and may not be moved. Consequently, one should not close the eyes of a person who has died, or straighten his limbs.

   Nevertheless, there are those who are accustomed to be lenient in this respect, and, in such a case, one should raise no objection, but, if possible, they should perform these activities with the aid of a non-*muktzeh* object which they hold, so that their hands should not come into direct contact with the dead body."[628]

2. *Shemirat Shabbat Kehilchatah* continues that on Shabbat, "One may tie a bandage round the head of the corpse, to prevent the jaw from opening wider, but 1) one should not tighten the bandage in such a way as to close the already open mouth and 2) one should beware not to tie a double knot."[629]

3. If the corpse must be transported to another part of the hospital on Shabbat via an elevator, someone who is not Jewish should transport the body and summon the elevator, but a Jew may accompany the corpse.[630]

4. When a body is transferred in a car on Shabbat by a driver who is not Jewish to a mortuary where someone designated to watch the body is waiting, it is not necessary to have a Jew watch over the body in the car for this short time [this concept is discussed in the next paragraph].

---

[627] R. Gavriel Goldman, *Min HaOlam V'ad HaOlam*, 55. This is for the honor of the deceased, so that they do not emit a foul odor. However, one may not violate Sabbath or festivals in order to provide air conditioning for a corpse, so it is advisable to use ice when there is no air conditioning available.

[628] *Shemirat Shabbat Kehilchatah* 64:8.

[629] Ibid.

[630] *Lev Avraham* 13:183; *Nishmat Avraham OH* 311:1 (6).

D. Post-Mortem Care

1a. It is customary to ensure that someone watches over the body from the time of death until the burial[631] as an expression of honor to the deceased and to protect the body.[632]

1b. When the body is in a generally safe place, it is permissible for the person who is watching over it to leave its presence for a short time,[633] such as when the nurses prepare the body to be discharged or one is needed to sign a death certificate or make funeral arrangements.

1c. If it is not possible to watch over the body in the same room, one should stand by the closest door outside of the room in which the deceased is being kept, and remain there.[634]

2. The body should not be washed by any hospital staff. However, any wound should be contained or covered to prevent flow of blood or any bodily fluids.

3. Any blood emitted from the body at the time of death is to be buried with the deceased. Consequently, one must ensure that:

   • All tubes (e.g., IV lines, gastric tubes, etc.) should be knotted as close to site as possible, cut above the knot and taped down in place.

   • Urinary catheters may be removed and discarded,[635] though it is best to leave catheters that are inserted into the body for the mortuary to remove.

   • No bandages or wound dressings should be removed.

   • If any blood is found on the clothing or linen of the deceased, it should be removed, inserted in a plastic bag, and placed in the body bag together with the deceased.

   • Amputated limbs are also often buried with the person, especially in cases of accidents presenting in the Emergency Department.

4. Although it is ideal for the mortuary to respectfully handle removal of all tubes, a patient who is intubated may be gently extubated by the hospital staff before the mortuary arrives in order to prevent disfiguration of the deceased's face.

5. Dentures should not be removed unless he or she made their wishes known beforehand to have them discarded. Prosthesis should also not be removed. If dentures or prostheses are not on the deceased at the time of death, they should be placed in a body bag for burial with the deceased. In most instances, they are buried together with the deceased.

---

[631] *Shulchan Aruch YD* 341:6.
[632] *Gesher Hachaim* 5:4 (4).
[633] *Igrot Moshe YD* 1:225.
[634] *Minhagim V'Kitzur Piskei Halachot Hanechutzot Al Kol Tzara Shelo Tavo*, Chevra Kaddisha Yitav Lev of Satmar, 5.
[635] *Lev Avraham* 13:179.

IX. Labor & Delivery

From about the time that the most intense phase of active labor begins, many traditionally observant couples observe a number of restrictions related to their physical interactions. These restrictions govern where in the room the husband may stand and prohibit the couple from touching one another, including hugging, kissing, or even passing the baby to each other, which is why they may ask a third party to pass the baby between them. Observance of these regulations should not be misunderstood as a lack of happiness or love between the couple.

1. Jewish law generally discourages medically inducing labor,[1] unless it must be done for a proper medical reason or to avoid other serious issues or problems.[2]

2. There are a number of blessings recited upon the birth of a child:

    • For a baby boy, both of the parents should recite the "*Hatov Ve'haMeitiv*" blessing immediately following the birth[3] (or as long as one still senses the joy of the birth).[4]

    • For a baby girl, both of the parents should recite the "*Shehecheyanu*" blessing the first time they see the baby[5] (or as long as one still senses the joy of the birth).[6]

    • For twins, in which there is a boy and a girl, the parents should only recite the "*Hatov Ve'haMeitiv*" blessing for both of the children.[7]

    • Once the mother has recovered from childbirth and feels that she has regained her strength, she can recite the "*Birkat HaGomel*" blessing with a Minyan.[8]

3. In a case of need, one may sign the name of their baby on a form, such as a birth certificate application, even before they have named their baby in the traditional manner, but they should only write the name down and not say it aloud.[9]

---

[1] *Igrot Moshe YD* 2:74 & 4:105; *Torat HaYoledet* 1:1-2. As a general rule the *Nishmat Avraham OH* 248:4 (1:2) writes that once a woman has reached the 42nd week of pregnancy she may take medication to induce labor but should do so early in the week if possible, so that she will not have to violate Shabbat (unless, of course, waiting presents any danger to the baby or the mother, in which case it should be done even on Shabbat).

[2] For example, one may induce in order to prevent danger to the mother or the baby but not simply for the sake of convenience. Preventing birth from taking place on Shabbat or a festival would not be a valid reason to induce, but having superior medical care may be.

[3] *Shulchan Aruch OH* 223:1.

[4] *Mishnah Berurah* 223:3.

[5] Ibid., 223:2. *Torat HaYoledet* 37:3.

[6] *Torat HaYoledet* 37:5.

[7] Ibid., 37:4.

[8] *Torat HaYoledet* 62:5; There are many different customs regarding making this blessing after childbirth. In some communities, women recite this blessing in the synagogue from the women's section after the Torah reading; in others, the blessing is said in the woman's home with a *Minyan*; others say it in the presence of other women and one man (*Mishnah Berurah* 119:3); while in many communities it is not customary for women to recite this blessing at all. See *Piskei Teshuvot* vol. 2, pg. 873-4, for a summary of the various customs and rabbinic opinions related to this matter. It is also possible for the husband to recite the blessing for his wife when he is called up to the Torah (*Mishnah Berurah* 119:17), though some discourage this practice (see the sources cited in *Nishmat Avraham OH* 119:(3)).

[9] *Otzar Habrit*, Rabbi Yosef David Weisberg, Jerusalem 1993, vol. 1 pg. 329. See also *Teshuvot V'Hanhagot* 3:297, who explains that there is a prophetical element to the parent's choice of a name, which is why it should not be shared before the *Brit* or naming because the listener's reaction might influence the parents to choose a different name,

4a.   If a baby boy is not medically stable enough to be circumcised on the eighth day, when he is customarily named as well, we wait until the circumcision is performed to give him a name.[10] However, if it is known that a significant period of time will pass before the circumcision can take place, many are accustomed to give the baby a name right away, even before the circumcision.[11]

4b.   If the parents are able to do so, it is customary when one has a baby boy whose circumcision will be delayed to nevertheless hold the *Shalom Zachar* on the first Friday night after birth, as is usually done, even if the baby was born on that Friday night.[12]

5.   See pages 51-56 for a discussion of issues related to labor and delivery, post-partum, the care of an infant, and nursing on Shabbat.

---

which had not been chosen under Divine inspiration. According to this reason, simply writing the name on a paper which will not be read by anyone in their presence should not be problematic. However, *Teshuvot V'Hanhagot* gives a second reason for not sharing a name until the *Brit*, which implies a connection between the soul of the baby and the occasion of the *Brit* so that it is better for the baby to receive the name only once he has been circumcised. According to this reason, we see why it is best to wait to share the name at all, if possible.

[10]   *Otzar Habrit* vol. 1 pg. 331.

[11]   *Nishmat Avraham YD* 263:2 (7) says in the name of *Rav Neuwirth* that if the circumcision will be delayed more than two weeks, the baby should be named before the *Brit*. Many are accustomed to name the baby beforehand only if the delay will be very lengthy, which frequently occurs with baby boys who have a condition known as hypospadias, for example, who often can't be circumcised until he is nearly a year old. Nevertheless, others—such as many Chassidim—always wait until the circumcision to name the child no matter how long it takes, unless he is the mother's firstborn child, in which case some have the practice of giving the name at the *Pidyon Haben* (*Otzar Habrit* vol. 1 pg. 331).

[12]   *Nishmat Avraham YD* 266:11 (8). On the other hand, it is reported that Rav Moshe Feinstein ruled that the *Shalom Zachar* should be held the Shabbat before the circumcision, and not the first Shabbat after the baby was born (*Sefer Mesoras Moshe*, pg. 353 fn. 336).

Rabbi Avrohom Friedlander

1157 Fifty First Street
Brooklyn, NY 11219
718-436-1089

אברהם יהושע העשיל פריעדלאנדער
●
אבד"ק היבנוב
רב דבית החולים מיימונידעס. בארא פארק
מחבר ספר חסדי אברהם. החולה בהלכה
ברוקלין. ניו יארק יע"א

בעזה"י

היום יום ראשון לסדר והסיר ה' **ממך כל חולי וגו'** (עקב), י"ד לחודש מנחם אב, יו"ד דרבה וקדישא של כ"ק מרן אא"ז הרה"ק רבן של ישראל מאוה"ג בעל אך פרי תבואה מליסקא זצוק"ל זי"ע ועכי"א, שנת **יבר"ך ישרא"ל** (תשע"ג) לפ"ק

הנה בא לפני הרה"ג איש כביר המעשה ר' **יהודה לייב וינער** הי"ו העוסק בצרכי ציבור באמונה לעזור ולהושיע אחינו בני ישראל המוטלים על ערש דוי ל"ע בבית החולים בעיר לאס אנדזשעליס יצ"ו, אשר יום ולילה לא ישבתו להקל מעליהם בעת צרתם, ובידידו קונטרס אשר זכה לחבר חיבור נחוץ ומועיל הנכתב בשפת המדינה בלשון ענגלי"ש, אשר כשמו כן הוא **"מדריך לחולים הנמצאים בבית החולים"**, והוא אוצר בלום ליקוטי הלכות ודינים והערות בדברים הנוגעים לכל עניני בית החולים, הן ברפואות והן לגבי התנהגות החולים הלכה למעשה כאו"א לפי מצבו, הן מה שנוגע לכשרות ושמירת המצות בעת חליים, ורוצה לאדפוסי אידרא, וביקש מאתי לעבור על הספר ולהשית עין עיוני בו, ואף כי בודאי קשה לי לומר שדעתי מסכמת עם כל מסקנותיו כי לא היה סיפק בידי לעמוד על כל דבריו, עכ"ז נתתי שמחה בלבי לראות שדבר יפה עשה בעטנו, וניכר בזה פרי עמלו ואיך מתמסר בעבודתו הקודש לעזור להחולים, ובלי ספק יפקו הימנו תועלת מרובה היושבים על מדין לדלות הימנו תיכף ומיד בלי שיהיו לחפש אחר עיון בזה, ושלא נהיה ח"ו נהיה הרי זה שופך דמים.

וע"כ אף ידי תיכון עמו להעלות ספרו על מכבש הדפוס ולהפיצו בישראל, ויהוד"ה אתה יודוך אחיך, ואמינא לפעלא טבא איישר חילא, ויעזור השי"ת שיוכל לברך על המוגמר לזכות ולהנות בו את הרבים ולהמשיך בעבודתו הקודש בפעולותיו בכלל ובפרט, וה' הטוב ישלח רפואה שלימה לכל חולי עמו ישראל, ובמהרה יקויים מאה"כ (ירמי') כי אעלה ארוכה לך וממכותיך ארפאך נאום ה', ונזכה להרמת קרן התורה וקרן ישראל בביאת גואל צדק במהרה בימינו אמן.

ולמען תת אות שעברתי על דפי הספר הנני אציין כמה הערות שנתעוררו אצלי, במה שהבאת בדף 44 מספר a3 בשם הגאון הגרש"ז אויערבאך ז"ל הובא דברי בשמירת שבת כהלכתה חלק ב' דף ל"ד, שהמדליק נרות לכבוד שב"ק בבית החולים בנר עלעקטארי הדלוק בכח בעטארי המיוחדין לנר של שבת יברך עליה, וגם אנכי הבאתי דברי בספרי חסדי אברהם ח"א בפרק ו' הלכות הדלקת נר של שבת ס"ג בהערה ו', עכ"ז ראה מש"כ שם מה שעוורר לי הגאון הצדיק קשש"ת רבי יחזקאל ראטה שליט"א אבד"ק קארלסבורג שמהשכנו להדליק בלא ברכה לצאת ידי כל הספיקות, ורק יכוון ויאמר בפירוש שמדליקות נרות אלו לכבוד שבת, וראה שם מש"כ בהערה ז', ודו"ק.

ומש"כ בדף 50 מספר 3b דבשבת ויו"ט, כשהמאכלים המבושלים מע"ש מתחממים ע"י אינם יהודים לצורך החולים, האם מותר לקרוביהם וכדומה לאכול ג"כ מהמאכלים הללו או לא, ראה בהאי ענינא בספרי חסדי אברהם ח"א במדור שאלות ותשובות שדנתי בזה באריכות עם גדולי פוסקי זמנינו, יעו"ש.

כ"ד ידידו ומעריצו, ומוקיר אני את פעולותיו הברוכים למען חולי עמך בית ישראל, אשר אין להאריך גודל המצוה כי רבה היא.

אברהם יהושע העשיל פריעדלאנדער
אבדק"ק היבנוב יצ"ו

Bibliography

Some of the contemporary works cited frequently in this booklet include:

Hebrew

- Auerbach, Rav Shlomo Zalman. *Shulchan Shlomo, Erchei Refuah.* Edited by Rabbi Simcha Bonem Lazerson. Jerusalem, Israel: 2005.

- Auerbach, Rav Shlomo Zalman. *Shulchan Shlomo, Hilchot Shabbat.* Edited by Rabbi Simcha Bonem Lazerson. Jerusalem, Israel: 1998.

- Avraham, Dr. Avraham S. *Lev Avraham.* 2nd edition. Jerusalem, Israel: Feldheim Publishers, 2009.

- Avraham, Dr. Avraham S. *Nishmat Avraham.* 2nd edition. Jerusalem, Israel: 2007.

- Friedlander, Rabbi Avraham. *Chasdei Avraham.* Brooklyn, NY: 1994.

- Lazerson, Rabbi Simcha Bonem. *B'shvilei Beit Harefuah.* Jerusalem, Israel: 2009.

- Zilberstein, Rav Yitzchak. *Torat HaYoledet.* B'nei B'rak, Israel: *Machon Halachah U'Refuah*, 1987.

- When the *Shemirat Shabbat Kehilchatah* is quoted, chapters 1-41 refer to the 2010 3rd edition, and chapters 42-68 refer to the 1989 edition, although when English quotes are taken directly from the *Shemirat Shabbat Kehilchatah*, it refers to the 1989 English edition published by Feldheim.

English

- Bodner, Rabbi Yisroel Pinchas, and Rabbi Daniel Roth, MD. *Halachos of Refuah on Shabbos.* Jerusalem, Israel: Feldheim Publishers, 2008.

- Handler, Rabbi Mechel, and Rabbi Dovid Weinberger. *Madrich L'chevra Hatzalah: A Digest of Halachos Pertaining to Pikuach Nefesh.* Jerusalem, Israel: Feldheim Publishers, 2008.

- Ribiat, Rabbi Dovid. *The 39 Melochos: An Elucidation of the 39 Melochos from Concept to Practical Application.* Jerusalem, Israel: Feldheim Publishers, 2001.

- Schachter, Rabbi Nachman. *Guide to Halachos.* Vol. 2. Third Edition. Edited and approved by Rabbi Moshe Heinemann. Jerusalem, Israel: Feldheim Publishers 2007.

- Weinberger, Rabbi Dovid. *Guide for the Jewish Hospital Patient.* New York City: Orthodox Union, 2011.

Index

www.ingramcontent.com/pod-product-compliance
Lightning Source LLC
LaVergne TN
LVHW051700080426

835511LV00017B/2652